Fasting – Cleanses, Renews and Rejuvenates

Bragg

THE MIRACLE OF
FASTING

PROVEN THROUGH HISTORY
For Physical, Mental and Spiritual Rejuvenation

PAUL C. BRAGG, N.D., Ph.D.
LIFE EXTENSION SPECIALIST
and
PATRICIA BRAGG, N.D., Ph.D.
HEALTH & FITNESS EXPERT

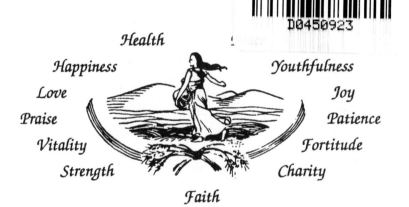

Health

Happiness   Youthfulness

Love   Joy

Praise   Patience

Vitality   Fortitude

Strength   Charity

Faith

JOIN
Bragg Health Crusades for a 100% Healthy World for All!

HEALTH SCIENCE
Box 7, Santa Barbara, California 93102 USA

World Wide Web: http://www.bragg.com

Notice: Our writings are to help guide you to live a healthy lifestyle and prevent health problems. If you suspect you have a medical problem, please seek alternative health professionals to help you make the healthiest informed choices. Diabetics should fast only under a health professional's supervision! If hypoglycemic, add Spirulina or barley green powder to liquids when fasting.

BRAGG

THE MIRACLE OF
FASTING

PAUL C. BRAGG, N.D., Ph.D.
LIFE EXTENSION SPECIALIST
and
PATRICIA BRAGG, N.D., Ph.D.
HEALTH & FITNESS EXPERT

Health Science, Box 7, Santa Barbara, California, 93102
Telephone (805) 968-1020, FAX (805) 968-1001

**To see Bragg Books and Products on-line,
visit our Web Site: http://www.bragg.com
e-mail address: bragg@bragg.com**

Quantity Purchases: Companies, Professional Groups, Churches, Clubs, Fundraisers etc. Please contact our Special Sales Department.

This book is printed on recycled, acid-free paper.

- REVISED AND EXPANDED -
Copyright © Health Science

Forty-seventh printing MCMXCVIII
ISBN: 0-87790-036-1

Published in the United States

HEALTH SCIENCE, Box 7, Santa Barbara, California 93102 USA

DEDICATION
We dedicate this Book to 8 Great Pioneers of Health and Longevity

Dr. August Rollier, M.D. –
Father of Heliotherapy (Sunshine Therapy)

Bernarr Macfadden –
Father and Founder of the Physical Culture Movement

Prof. Arnold Ehret –
Originator of the Mucusless Diet Healing System

Dr. St. Louis Estes, D.D.S. –
One of the greatest, dynamic Nutrition Speakers

Dr. Benedict Lust, M.D. –
Father and Founder of Naturopathy in America

Dr. John Harvey Kellogg, M.D. –
Director for 60 years of the Battle Creek Health Sanitarium in Battle Creek, Michigan

Dr. Henry Lindlahr, M.D. –
Famous Drugless Physician, who pioneered the return to Natural Methods of Treatment

Dr. John T. Tilden, M.D. –
Great Natural Healer and Health Pioneer

Patricia Bragg   *Paul C. Bragg*

Fasting Helps Keep You Healthy & Youthful

Fasting is an effective and safe method of detoxifying the body – a technique that wise men have used for centuries to heal the sick. Fast regularly and help the body heal itself and stay well. Give all of your organs a rest. Fasting can help reverse the ageing process, and if we use it correctly, we will live longer, happier lives. Just three days a month will do it. Each time you complete a fast, you will feel better. Your body will have a chance to heal and rebuild its immune system by regular fasting. You can fight off illness and the degenerative diseases so common in this chemically polluted environment we live in. When you feel a cold or any illness coming on, or are just depressed – it's best to fast!

– James Balch, M.D., *Prescription for Nutritional Healing*
"Bragg books were my conversion to the healthy way."

i

BRAGG HEALTH CRUSADES for the 21st CENTURY
Teaching People Worldwide to Live
Healthier, Stronger Lives for a Better World

We love sharing, teaching and giving, and you can share this love by being a partner with Bragg Health Crusades World-Wide Outreach. Bragg Crusades is dedicated to helping others! We feel blessed when your life improves through following our teachings from the Bragg Books and Crusades. It makes all our years of faithful service so worthwhile!

The Miracle of Fasting book has been the #1 book for 13 years in Russia! Why? Because we show them how to live a healthy, wholesome life for less money, and it's so easy to understand and follow. Most healthful lifestyle habits are free (eg. - good posture, clean thoughts, plain natural foods, exercise and deep breathing, that draws energy into the body). We continue to reach the multitudes with all our health teachings, lectures, Crusades, radio, TV and video outreaches.

My joy and priorities come from God and healthy living. I'm excited about spreading health worldwide, for now it's needed more than ever! My father and I also pioneered Health TV with our program "Health and Happiness" filmed in Hollywood. It's thrilling to be a Health Crusader and you will enjoy it also. See back pages to list names (yourself, family, friends) who you think would like to receive our free Health Bulletins!

By reading Bragg Self-Health Books you gain a new confidence that you can help yourself, family and friends to Healthy Principles of Living! Please call your local health store and book store and ask for the Bragg Health Books. Prayerfully, we hope to have all stores stock the Bragg Books so they will be available to everyone.

I have visions of **Health Retreats** where people can find joyous health and rebirth! They will be **Recharging - Physically, Mentally, Emotionally and Spiritually.** Everyone needs retreats now, more than ever!

For the new millennium, we are planning Bragg Recharge Retreats and Child & Senior Care Centers which are desperately needed across America. We are just waiting for the right locations and funding. We can accept all gifts, monetary and land (appraised value), and we can give a receipt for tax deductions. Seldom-used ranches, farms and old estates could become Recharge Centers for rejuvenating mind, body and soul. Those attending would become health crusaders for their families and friends. Empty buildings and spacious older homes with yards would make ideal Child & Senior Centers. If you have a location and would like to be part of this great outreach, please call or write to me.

We are not new to retreats; I was reared on retreats. Holidays and vacations were spent at camp and retreats for precious weeks of growth and recharge. My Dad pioneered the first health spa (Macfadden's Deauville) in Miami Beach and others in Highland Springs, CA, and Danville, NY.

I expend all my energy and funds inspiring and helping others to help and heal themselves! Genuine love seeks ways to express itself! I thank you for your caring, sharing support – with your help we can achieve our future goals! I know God will bless you. Your needed help will be a blessing to The Bragg Health Crusades. Our budget is for a mighty worthwhile cause. I know you, your family and friends will enjoy and benefit from our teachings and health retreats.

With A Loving, Grateful Heart, *Patricia Bragg*

BRAGG HEALTH CRUSADES, America's Health Pioneers
A non-profit organization. Gifts are tax deductible.
7340 Hollister Ave., Santa Barbara, CA 93117 USA (805) 968-1020
Over 85 continuous years spreading health & fitness worldwide

ii

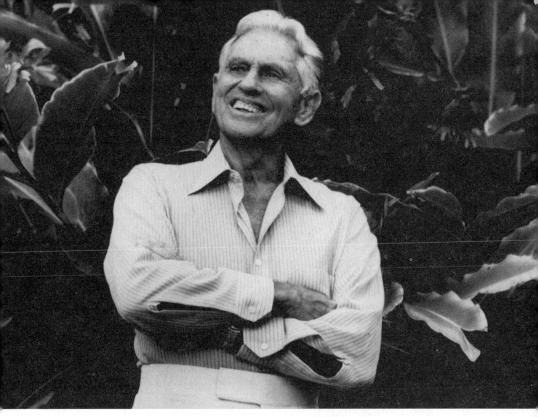

PAUL C. BRAGG, N.D., Ph.D.
World's Leading Healthy Lifestyle Authority

Paul C. Bragg's daughter Patricia and their wonderful, healthy members of the Bragg *Longer Life, Health and Happiness Club* exercise daily on the beautiful Fort DeRussy lawn, at world famous Waikiki Beach in Honolulu, Hawaii. Membership is free and open to everyone who wishes to attend any morning – Monday through Saturday, from 9 to 10:30 am – for Bragg Deep Breathing and health and fitness exercises. On Saturday there are often health lectures on how to live a long, healthy life! The group averages 75 to 125 per day, depending on the season. From December to March it can go up to 200. Its dedicated leaders have been carrying on the class for over 27 years. Thousands have visited the club from around the world and carried the Bragg health and fitness message to friends and relatives back home. When you visit Honolulu, Hawaii, Patricia invites you and your friends to join her and the club for wholesome, healthy fellowship. She also recommends you visit the outer Hawaiian Islands (Kauai, Hawaii, Maui, Molokai) for a fulfilling, healthy vacation.

To maintain good health, normal weight and increase the good life of radiant health, joy and happiness, the body must be exercised properly (stretching, walking, jogging, running, biking, swimming, deep breathing, good posture, etc.) and nourished wisely with natural foods. – Paul C. Bragg

iii

Fasting Cleanses, Renews and Rejuvenates

Our bodies have a natural self-cleansing for maintaining a clean, healthy body and our "river of life" – our blood. It's essential we keep our entire bodily machinery from head to toes healthy and in good working order so nothing breaks down!

Fasting is the best detoxifying method. It's also the most effective and safest way to increase elimination of waste buildups and enhance the body's miraculous self-healing and self-repairing process that keeps you healthy and youthful.

If you prepare for a fast by eating a cleansing diet for 1 to 2 days, this can greatly facilitate the cleansing process. Fresh variety salads and organic vegetables, fruits and their juices, as well as fruit pep drinks and green drinks (alfalfa, barley green, chlorella, spirulina, wheatgrass, etc.) stimulates waste elimination. Fresh foods and juices can literally pick up dead matter from your body and dispose of it. After pre-cleansing period start your fast.

Daily, even on most fast days, we take from 1,000 to 3,000 mg. of mixed vitamin C powder (C concentrate, acerola, rosehips and bioflavonoids) in liquids. It's a potent antioxidant and flushes out deadly free radicals. It also promotes collagen production for new healthy tissues. Vitamin C is important if you are detoxifying from prescription drugs or alcohol overload.

A moderate, well planned distilled water fast is our favorite or the introductory fast of diluted fresh juice (35% distilled water). Both can cleanse your body of excess mucus, old fecal matter, trapped cellular, non-food wastes and help remove inorganic mineral deposits and sludge from your pipes and joints.

Fasting works by self-digestion. During a fast your body intuitively will decompose and burn only the substances and tissues that are damaged, diseased or unneeded, such as abscesses, tumors, excess fat deposits, excess water and congestive wastes.

Even a short fast (1 to 3 days) will accelerate elimination from your liver, kidneys, lungs, bloodstream and skin. Sometimes you will experience dramatic changes (cleansing and healing crisis) as accumulated wastes are expelled. With your first fasts you may temporarily have cleansing headaches, fatigue, body odor, bad breath, coated tongue, mouth sores and even diarrhea as your body is cleaning house. Please be patient with your body!

After a fast your body begins to healthfully rebalance when you faithfully follow The Bragg Healthy Lifestyle. Your weekly 24 hour fast removes toxins on a regular basis, so they don't accumulate. Your energy levels will rise and shine – physically, mentally, emotionally and spiritually. Your creativity expands. You will feel like a "new you" – which you are – you are being cleansed, purified and reborn. Fasting is a miracle!

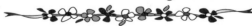

You are what you eat, drink, breathe, think and do! – Patricia Bragg

iv

THE MIRACLE OF FASTING

To preserve health is a moral and religious duty, for health is the basis for all social virtues. We can no longer be as useful when not well.
– Dr. Samuel Johnson,
Father of Dictionaries

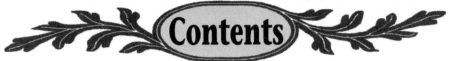

Contents

Chapter 1: The Miracle of Fasting 1
Helps You Enjoy a Super Charged, Healthy, Happy, Long Life 1
Bragg Motto – I Love Life and I Want to Live! 2
Unhealthy Lifestyle Killing Millions Worldwide! 2
Sickness is a Crime Against Your Body – Don't Be a Criminal 3
Life Can Be a Happy and Joyous Adventure 4

Chapter 2: What is the Miracle of Fasting? 5
What is the Most Significant Discovery of This Modern Age? 5
Fasting Conserves Energy – Your Vital Force 6
We Live in a Poisoned World 7
The Big, Filthy Sewer in the Sky Above Us 7
Rivers, Lakes & Oceans Becoming Polluted 8
Fasting – The Key to Internal Purification 9
Poisons from Chemical Pesticides & Sprays 9
Fasting Aids in Flushing Deadly Poisons from the Body 11
Health Menace – Waxed Fruits and Vegetables! 12
Synthetic, Toxic Food Additives Can Kill 14
Salt Causes Edema, Kidney Problems, etc. 16
What Salt Does to Your Blood Pressure 16
Why Cows are Given Large Amounts of Salt 17
Americans Are Salt-a-holics! 18
Death Valley Hike Proved Salt Dangerous 18
Fasting De-Salts Body Cells and Organs 22
Fasting is the Great Cleanser and Purifier 23
Do You Have Harmful Habits You Must Overcome? 25
Fasting – The Key to Super Energy 26
Fasting – A Natural Instinct and Great Purifier 27
Jesus, His Disciples and Many Great Teachers Fasted 28

Chapter 3: The Enemy Within Our Bodies 29
Rid Yourself of Depression 30
Unhealthy Lifestyle & Overeating are Killers 31
Why Not Enjoy Life to 120? 32
Outwit Acidosis that Affects Millions 34
Raw Fruits and Vegetables Are Mother Nature's Miracle Cleansers . . . 35
Your Mind Must Control Your Body 36
Perfect Balancer – Apple Cider Vinegar 38

When you sell a man a book you don't just sell him paper, ink and glue, you sell him a whole new life! There's heaven and earth in a real book. The real purpose of books is to inspire the mind into its own thinking. – Christopher Morley

v

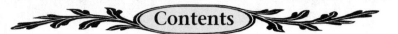

Contents

Chapter 4: Fasting Fights Deadly Acid Crystals 39

Toxic Acid Crystals Can Cement Your Joints to Make You Stiff 39
How Toxic Acid Crystals Build in Your Body 40
Back Pains – The Curse of Mankind 42
Fasting for Purification 43
Victory Won By Fasting, Diet and Exercise 44
Mother Nature Works Slowly, But Surely 45

Chapter 5: Scientific Fasting Explained 47

Fasting is as Old as Man 48
Fasting Awakens the Mind and Soul 49
The Biblical Patriarchs Fasted 50
Fasting – The Safe, Perfect Cleanser 51
Don't be a Slave to Food 51
Plan Your Fasting Program Today 52
Your Mind Must Rule Your Body to Fast Successfully 53
No Breakfast Plan is Best 53
Healthy Eating Habits Keep You Youthful 55
Americans Love to Eat Socially! 56
Keeping Internally Clean is Critical 56
Are You Ready to Fast, Detox and Get Healthy? 57
Juice Fast – an Introduction to Water Fast 58
Some Powerful Juice Combinations 59
The 70% Watery Human 60

Chapter 6: Why I Drink Only Distilled Water! 61

Hard Inorganic Minerals Cause Problems! 62
Millions Drink Rain (Distilled) Water 63
Distilled Water is Best for Your Health 64
Ten Reasons to Drink Distilled Water (list) 66

Chapter 7: How Long Should One Fast? 67

Shorter Fasts Are Better and Safer 68
Why Should You Fast? 69
Great Benefits From Short and Long Fasts 70
Fasting Appreciated Worldwide 71
Pre-Cleanse For Better Fasting Results 72
Here is My Fasting Program – Which I Recommend 73
Breaking Health Laws – You Pay the Price! 74

Chapter 8: How to Break a 24 Hour Fast 75

Follow These Instructions Carefully! 75
Your Kidneys – The Miracle Organs 75
A Swiss Doctor Was My Human Savior 76
Keep Your Meals Healthy and Simple 78
The Vegetarian Diet is Healthiest! 79

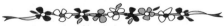

It is never too late to be what you might have been. – George Elliot

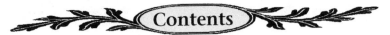

Contents

Chapter 9: I Fast 7 to 10 Days, 4 Times a Year **81**

Here's the Path to Perfect Health! .81
Fasting Balances Your Thermostat Naturally 82
Mother Nature Intended the Body and Breath to Be Sweet 83
Unhealthy Lifestyle Causes Chronic Fatigue 84
Fasting Pulls Out Toxins and Poisons 85
Fasting Promotes Healthy Elimination 87
How to Conduct a 3 Day, 7 Day & 10 Day Fast 88

Chapter 10: How to Break Long Fasts **89**

How to Break a 7 Day Fast 89
How to Break a 10 Day Fast 90
The Ideal Elimination Program .91
Vegetarianism Versus Meat Eating 92
Eliminating Meat is Safer & Healthier 94
Seven of My Beloved Teachers .95

Chapter 11: Your Tongue Never Lies **97**

The Body Can Take a Lot of Abuse 98
Learn to Read Your Tongue's Message 99

Chapter 12: Just Grin and Bear It **101**

Don't Live to Eat – Eat to Live & Be Healthy 102
Give the Vital Force a Chance to Clean House 103

Chapter 13: Fasting Fights and Removes Mucus **105**

American Diet Forms Mucus and Illness 106
Mucus Shows Up in the Urine when Fasting 107
Winter Miseries? Or Body Cleansing? 108
Take the Mucus Test 109
Breaking Bad Habits Through Fasting 110
Deadly Smoking Facts! (list) 112

Chapter 14: Fasting Melts Away Pounds! **113**

Fat is a Burden and Health Risk! 114
Fasting Rewards You with Increased Energy 115
Your Waistline is Your Lifeline & Dateline! 116
Fasting – A Challenge to Improve Your Health & Looks 117
Do These Exercises Daily 118

Chapter 15: How to Gain Weight by Fasting **119**

Miracles Happen With Fasting! .122
Fasting is a Weight Normalizer .123
The Doctor of the Future (graphic) 123

*Open thou mine eyes, that I may behold
wondrous things out of thy law. – Psalms 119:18*

Men do not die, they kill themselves. – Seneca, Roman Philosopher

Contents

Chapter 16: Fasting Fights Winter Miseries **125**
Fast and Rest For Your Healing! 126
The Body is Self-Healing & Self-Repairing 127
Premature Ageing (graphic) 128

Chapter 17: Outwit Premature Ageing **129**
Take This Quiz and The Mirror Test 129
Recharged, So at 70 World Tennis Champ 131
The Opportunity of Your Lifetime 132

Chapter 18: Fasting Keeps the Arteries Young **133**
You are as Old as Your Arteries 134
Shocking Heart Facts About the #1 Killer 134
What You Eat and Drink Becomes You 135
Eat Healthy – Live Healthy – Live Long 136
The Heart and Circulatory System (graphic) 137
Healthy Heart Habits For a Long, Vital Life (chart) 138
Recommended Blood Chemistry Values 138

You Have Nine Doctors at Your Command **139**

Chapter 19: Doctor Sunshine **141**
Sunshine Brings Peace, Relaxation to Nerves 142
Gentle Sun Rays are Soothing and Best 143

Chapter 20: Doctor Fresh Air **145**
Our Body is a Breathing Machine 146
Deep Breathers Live Longer 147
India's Holy Men Practice Deep, Slow Breathing 148
Deep Breathing – Secret of Endurance 149

Chapter 21: Doctor Pure Water **153**
The Water You Drink Can Make or Break Your Health! 153
Most Ancient Healers Used Water Therapy 154
How Our Body Uses Water 156

Chapter 22: Doctor Good Natural Food **165**
Healthy Foods Build and Maintain Your Body! 166
Iodine from Kelp is Important 169
The Effect of Good Food on the Brain 169
Alcohol, Toxins and Drugs Are Killers! 170
Refined, Processed Foods Produce Learning Disabled Children . . .170
Most Young American Men Are Unfit 171
American Adults are in a Sad Physical & Mental Condition 173
Mental, Physical and Spiritual Rewards 174
Healthy Eating is a Science! 175

*We can no more afford to spend major time on minor things,
than we can to spend minor time on major things! – Jim Rohn*

Contents

Chapter 23: Doctor Fasting **177**

Chapter 24: Doctor Exercise **179**

The Major Muscles of the Human Body (graphic) 180
Exercise Normalizes Blood Pressure 181
Walking for Health , Fitness and Life 181
Walking – The King of Exercise 182
The Importance of Abdominal Exercises 183
Should You Exercise While Fasting? 183
Iron Pumping Oldsters 185
Amazing Strength Results in 8 Weeks 186
Study Shows Fitness Improves Wellness 186
Paul Bragg LIfting Weights (photo)

Chapter 25: Doctor Rest **189**

Check Your Mattress (graphic) 190
Why Do We Rest? 190
Rest Must Be Earned 191
Life is Meant to be Enjoyed, Not Hectic & Rushed 192
Mother Nature Knows What's Best! 193
Relax and Enjoy Your Life – It's No Crime 194
Some Relaxation Techniques 195
Insomnia Will Vanish 196

Chapter 26: Doctor Good Posture **197**

Posture Chart (graphic) 197
Take the Mirror Posture Test 198
Bragg Posture Exercise 198
Good Posture is Important For Health 200
How to Sit, Stand and Walk for Strength, Youthfulness, Health . .200
Illness That Cannot Be Cured By Fasting, Cannot Be Cured 202

Chapter 27: Doctor Human Mind **203**

Brain Areas (graphic) 203
Your Body, Your Precious Home – Protect It 204
Correct Thinking Important for Health 204
Your Mind Must Control Your Body! 205
Drugs Control Addict's Mind! 205
Let Your Mind Guide You to Health! 207
Miracle Rewards With Fasting 207
Inner Spiritual Harmony is Important 208

Kindness should be a frame of mind in which we are alert to every opportunity: to do, to give, to share and to cheer. – Patricia Bragg

Nature cannot be hastened. The bloom of a flower opens in its own proper time. – Paul Bruton

The head is clearer, the health is better, the heart is lighter and the purse is heavier. – Scottish clergyman on fasting, circa 1800.

ix

Contents

Chapter 28: Spiritual Aspects of Fasting 209

Fasting Gives Mental & Physical Awareness 210
Great Spiritual Leaders Practiced Fasting 211
My Unforgettable Experience with Gandhi 211
Fasting Brings Spiritual Rebirth to All Who Cleanse 213
The Grotto Where Jesus Fasted 213
The Fast of 40 Days and 40 Nights 214
A Sound Mind in a Sound Body 215
Your Body is Your Temple and Needs the Best Care 216
Take Time for 12 Things (list) 217
The Bragg Healthy Lifestyle 218

Chapter 29: The Science of Eating For Super Health ... 219

A Tropical Paradise for Health 220
Eat Simple and Natural to Stay Healthy 224
Organic Fruits – the Prize Food of Man (list) 225
Nut and Seed List 225
Organic Vegetables – The Purifiers and Protectors 226
Natural Sweetening Agents 227
Natural Oils 227
Natural Whole Grains, Flours and Cereals 227
Sample Health Menus 228
Healthy Beverages (recipes) 230
The Bragg Pep Drink 230
Vegetable Protein Percentage (chart) 233
Foods Naturally Rich in Vitamin E (chart) 234
Phytochemicals Help Prevent Cancer (chart) 235
Body Signs of Potassium Deficiency (chart) 236
Avoid These Processed, Refined, Harmful Foods (list) 237
The Miracles of Apple Cider Vinegar (list) 238

Chapter 30: Mother Nature Knows No Mercy 239

Mother Nature Wants Us Clean & Healthy 240
Which Kind of Person are You? 240
Alternative Health Therapies 241-244
Boron – Miracle Trace Mineral for Healthy Bones 245
Miraculous Testimonials 246-248
Index 249-251

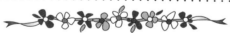

*Living in harmony with the universe is living
totally alive, full of vitality, health, joy, power, love,
and abundance on every level. – Shakti Gawain*

Nature never makes any fuss, and yet it does everything. – Lao-tzu

On a fast day you shall read the words of the Lord. – Jeremiah 36:6

*If I were to name the three most precious resources of life, I would
say books (Bible, etc.), friends and nature; and the greatest, the most
constant and always at hand is nature. – John Burroughs*

Fasting Brings Great Health Miracles!

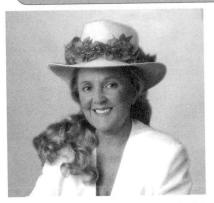

Patricia Bragg is a genuine Health Crusader like her father and is a living example of The Bragg Healthy Lifestyle. She speaks at conventions, schools, colleges, churchs, prisons and seminars throughout the world.

Throughout history and in the Bible, fasting has long been promoted as a spiritual means for intensifying prayer and your faith. You can reap great spiritual blessings with your fasting and prayer. Those who knew the secrets and the great benefits of fasting as a vital dimension in God include Jesus, the Apostle Paul, the early church leaders, Daniel, Elijah, Ezra, Esther, Job, David, Hannah, Isaiah, Zachariah and others. Prominent fasters in the annals of Christian history include John Calvin, Martin Luther, John Knox, John Wesley, David Brainard, George Muller, and hundreds of other church pioneers.

They discovered that abstaining from food not only freed them to focus upon God with fresh intensity, but also opened avenues of spiritual perception and understanding that were not available during routine living. They found as they focused upon God with deliberate discipline and prayer, God focused upon them with clarity of direction and quickening of spirit. They could partake of God more easily when all else was set aside. Fasting Brings Great Spiritual, Mental, Emotional and Physical Health Miracles!

A teacher for the day can be a guiding light for a lifetime!
Bragg Books are silent health teachers – never tiring, ready night or day to help you help yourself to health! Our books are written with love and a deep desire to guide you to healthy lifestyle living. – Patricia Bragg

The freedom and ease you experience during fasting enables you to discover new undreamed of depths to the meaning of life. – Herbert Shelton

Don't procrastinate and keep waiting for "the right moment." Today – take action and plan, plot and follow through with your goals, dreams and healthy lifestyle living! You will be a winner in life when you Captain your life to success!
– Patricia Bragg

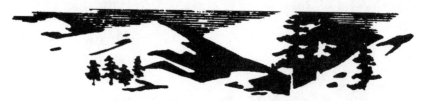

TEN HEALTH COMMANDMENTS

Thou shall respect and protect thy body as the highest manifestation of life.

Thou shall abstain from all unnatural, devitalized food and stimulating beverages.

Thou shall nourish thy body with only Natural unprocessed, live foods, that . . .

Thou shall extend thy years in health for loving, sharing with others and charitable service.

Thou shall regenerate thy body by the right balance of activity and rest.

Thou shall purify thy cells, tissues and blood with healthy foods, pure water, fresh air and sunshine.

Thou shall abstain from all food when out of sorts in mind or body.

Thou shall keep all thoughts, words and emotions pure, good, calm, kind, uplifting and loving.

Thou shall increase thy knowledge of Nature's Laws, follow them and enjoy the fruits of thy life's labor.

Thou shall lift up thyself, friends and family by obedience to God's Healthy, Pure Laws of Living.

Paul C. Bragg   Patricia Bragg

And Jesus full of the Holy Ghost returned from Jordan and was lead by the Spirit into the wilderness. Jesus fasted for 40 days and when the fast was ended He afterward hungered. – Luke 4:1-2

Bragg Healthy Lifestyle Plan

- *Read, plan, plot and follow through for supreme health and longevity.*
- *Organizing your lifestyle helps you identify what's important in your life.*
- *Where space allows we have included "words of wisdom" from great minds to motivate and inspire you.*
- *Underline, highlight or dog-ear pages as you read important passages.*
- *Be faithful to your health goals everyday for a healthy, strong, happy life.*

Chapter 1

The Miracle of Fasting

Helps You Enjoy a Super Charged, Healthy, Happy Long Life

Every thinking person must at one time or another say to himself, "Am I getting the most out of life?" The great comedian, Ed Wynn said, "Without your health, riches, possessions and fame are all mud." What is a man without health, even though endowed with riches and fame? Riches cannot buy health and happiness. Just because a person has achieved fame, it does not follow that he is healthy and happy!

I do not discredit success and riches! I think money and possessions have a place in our lives. Physical comforts and luxuries are important to most people. Take away a man's wealth and give him only health and his first desire will be the return of his riches.

But with both achieved, a word remains which we hate to utter; a thought we dread to contemplate; a thing which gives sorrow, pain and grief. That word, that thought, that thing, is death! Even in cases where life appears a burden, how tenaciously does man cling to it! How the spirit recoils from a struggle with death! How fondly it retains its grasp on life! Man's great desire is for health and long life on earth; "Man clings to the world as his home, and would want to live here forever, if he had health and long-lasting youthfulness."

Note: *My father and I wrote this book together. However, because my father is both my mentor and the American Pioneer of Fasting – with long years of experience overseeing the fasting of thousands of students with miraculous results – this text is mostly presented in his voice.* – Patricia Bragg

"Yet even now", says the Lord, "return to me with all your heart, with fasting." – Joel 2:12

Bragg Motto – I Love Life and I Want to Live!

At our Bragg Health Crusade lectures, I often sing my favorite song – called "I Love Life, and I Want to Live"– for my students. These strong words express the inner desires of each one of us. Life in itself is a miracle! And you and I who have precious life are holding this miracle in the palms of our hands to treasure and protect.

Life is Precious – It's the Treasure of Treasures

Since Adam and Eve lived in that historic Garden of Eden, the prolongation of human life has been and still is mankind's biggest challenge! The Persian and Greek sages, in the centuries before Christ, summoned their intellectual forces to solve it in vain. The scholars of the Medieval Ages pursued it zealously, but again were stymied. Today, in this fast-paced space age, every intelligent person deep in their heart and soul wants to live a healthy, long life. Most lack the proper health knowledge – the true key to a long, active, healthy life!

By following my mentors – Mother Nature's and God's Natural Laws, I invented the Bragg Healthy Lifestyle. Follow it and you can live to a healthy, active, advanced age! Every person owes it to himself, his relatives, his friends and his country to take care of his health! This will make him a valued, active citizen, not a financial burden! I believe that every one is entitled to active lives of 120 years or more as the Bible states,

"Man's days shall be 120 years." – Genesis 6:3

Longevity may be defined as the maximum duration of life that a healthy person can attain under the most healthy, favorable conditions by living a healthy lifestyle.

Unhealthy Lifestyle Killing Millions Worldwide!

Most people – because of their unwise habits in diet, drink and excesses – die prematurely, long before fulfilling their potential. Wild animals, undisturbed, live out their full term. Man's the only exception. Sadly, not more than one in a million lives out his natural life.

If you would imitate Nature, you should take her simplicity for your model.
– M. Sendibogius

Sickness is a Crime Against Your Body – Don't Be a Health Criminal!

Animals in their wild habitat know by instinct how to live, and what to eat and drink. They know how to fast by natural instinct when they get hurt or sick. Naturally, animals are led to eat what is good for them. But man eats and drinks anything and everything – consuming the most indigestible concoctions, washing it down with poisonous slops – and then wonders why he is sickly and does not live to be a centenarian!

In theory, humans desire long life! Many shorten their lives to the minimum. Does this make sense? Why this marvelous mechanism of man – perfect in its minutest organism, combining a Godlike intelligence with a body which sculptors have imitated but never equalled – should be ruthlessly destroyed by its owner's unhealthy lifestyle is one of the inexplicable disgraces of our culture!

The world famous marble statue of Apollo that Patricia and I saw in the Vatican at Rome is not greater in the perfection of manly beauty than that possessed by thousands of young men in our midst today. This inanimate marble of Apollo is as tenderly cared for as a rare, priceless jewel. Meanwhile, living man – noble, intellectual, refined, with a miraculous physical structure and an eternal soul – gives his wonderful body less attention than he gives to his car, cat or dog.

All people of sound mentality naturally desire a long, healthy, pain-free, happy and useful life. With our natural intelligence – super health, happiness and longevity should be the rule instead of the exception.

In my early career, I was associated with the great Bernarr Macfadden, the Father and Founder of the Physical Culture movement. I was the associate Editor of the pioneer health magazine *Physical Culture*. These lines always appeared on the front cover of every issue:

> **"Sickness is a crime – Don't be a criminal."**

Old age is a highly toxic condition caused by nutritional deficiencies and an unhealthy lifestyle.

Physical weakness, flabbiness and sickness have always seemed criminal to me – a sacrilegious abuse of that miracle instrument, the human body. I regained my health after being a hopeless tuberculosis victim years ago, and since then I've made a religion of keeping in perfect health through conscientious care of my body. Adhering to a high ideal of stamina, vitality, health and endurance has paid me great dividends – so priceless that I call myself "A Health Billionaire!"

> **To Be a Health Billionaire and Enjoy the Glow of Ageless Health and Happiness, You Must Work for It!**

The "secret" of the glow of ageless health lies in maintaining internal cleanliness and regeneration. This requires eating natural, organically grown live foods, combined with other healthy practices such as fasting, drinking distilled water, exercising and deep breathing.

When you purify your body with systematic fasting and live foods, you crave daily exercise. And by exercising you sculpt your body to become the person you want to be. Just think, from this minute on you can mold your body to physical perfection. With the knowledge found in these pages you will find out how you can reap the most out of life, physically, mentally and spiritually!

The human race is a unique study, and an intriguing one! But the natural laws which govern man are simple and understandable if one takes the time to learn and observe how he functions from day to day!

Life Can Be a Happy and Joyous Adventure

To know one's self seems like an endless task, but with crystal clear observation and the daily application of these simple but precise laws, life becomes not only a most exciting adventure, but a tremendous joy! Study and follow The Bragg Healthy Lifestyle throughout your life, and you will start to experience the day-by-day joys, happiness and truly great pleasures of a healthy body, mind and soul for a happy, long and vigorous life!

Instead of medicine, fast for a day. – Plutarch, Greek Philosopher

Chapter 2

What is *The Miracle of Fasting?*

What is the Most Significant Discovery of this Modern Age?

- The finding of Dinosaur eggs on the plains of Mongolia, which scientists assert were laid some 10,000,000 years ago?
- The unearthing of ancient tombs and cities, with their confirmations of the Scriptural stories, and their matchless specimens of bygone civilizations?
- The radioactive time clock by which Professor Lane of Tufts University estimates the age of the earth as 1,250,000,000 years?
- Jet airplanes? Space travel? Lasers? Television? Radio? Computers? Telephones? Cell phones? Automobiles?

(None of the above compare with fasting . . .)

5

The Greatest Discovery of Modern Times

In our opinion, the greatest discovery by modern man is the method to rejuvenate himself physically, mentally and spiritually by fasting. Man can create a quality of agelessness and with fasting, can prevent premature ageing and a premature death!

The dread of "growing old" and becoming a burden to himself and others is one of man's greatest fears. The fear of becoming sick, senile, helpless and unable to care for one's self is rooted deep in every thinking person's mind. With the complete knowledge of fasting and The Bragg Healthy Lifestyle, as outlined in this book, you can banish all your fears of premature ageing! With a 24 hour complete water fast weekly – setting aside 52 days and four 7 to 10 day fasts a year for body purification – you can keep the toxins removed and flush the rust and crystals from your moveable joints and muscles. You

---

I have found a perfect health, a new state of existence, a feeling of purity and happiness, something unknown to humans!
– Novelist Upton Sinclair, a frequent faster

must bear in mind that it is the toxic debris and wastes of metabolism (from the biological process of converting food into living matter and the matter into energy) that brings on many physical ailments and premature ageing.

When the Vital Force of your body drops below normal, then all your physical problems – as well as your mental ones – begin! Read the Bragg *Build Powerful Nerve Force* Book. (See back pages for booklist.) It details how to reduce stress, fear, anger and worry – these negative factors can destroy your precious Vital Force and life!

Fasting Conserves Energy – Your Vital Force

Let me explain. We eat food and as it passes through the body, it must be masticated, digested, assimilated and then the waste is eliminated. We have four great organs of elimination: the bowels, the kidneys, the lungs, and the skin. In order for these eliminative organs to work perfectly, the body must build a high Vital Force of body energy reserves.

It takes a tremendous amount of Vital Force to pass a large meal through the gastrointestinal tract and also eliminate the waste via the 30 foot tube that runs from the mouth to the rectum. It takes the great power of Vital Force to pass liquids through the 2 million filters of the human kidneys. It takes Vital Force for the chemical power of the liver and the gallbladder to do their work in preparing food for the billions of body cells. It takes great Vital Force for the lungs to deeply inhale up to 2 quarts of oxygen with each breath, to purify the entire bloodstream in your body and expel the toxins and the carbon dioxide. It takes great Vital Force for the skin (often called your third kidney) with its 96 million pores, to throw off body toxins in the form of skin rashes, pimples, sweat and foul body odors.

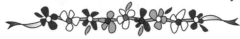

The Endless Quest
Freedom and progress rest in man's continual search for truth.
Truth is the summit of being. – Emerson

Who is strong? He that can conquer his bad habits. – Ben Franklin

We Live in a Poisoned World

It is the duty of your Vital Force to supply the energy used to rid the body of any toxins created during the processing of food consumed. The Vital Force must also keep the body temperature at 98.6 degrees. When sick the body will often create a fever to burn up the toxins to flush them out! If it falls below this figure you are enervated and sick. In our modern civilization, the Vital Force is becoming so overburdened with toxic filth, pollution and toxins in foods that man keeps creating.

The Big, Filthy Sewer in the Sky Above Us

We are bombarded with noxious and harmful filth and dirt from our skies. Take New York City as an example. Roughly 60 tons of airborne dust particles fall monthly on each square mile. Think of all the airborne dirt the body must battle with to keep a person in New York alive! No wonder there are so many hospitals and sick people in that poisoned, toxic city.

Scientists estimate that an inhabitant of an industrial city such as Pittsburgh, Pennsylvania or Birmingham, Alabama stands a higher than average chance of contracting a deadly lung disease or suffering from heart trouble, just because of breathing polluted air. That special form of poisoned air known as "smog" regularly affects not only Los Angeles, but Phoenix, St. Louis, Kansas City, Washington, D.C., New York City and most big cities across America as well as around the world.

A grim mixture of soot and smoke from factories, incinerators and power plants; the gaseous by-products of industry; and the toxic exhaust from cars and trucks are making an ugly, unhealthy mess out of the air most Americans breathe. Air pollution is a real menace to our health and lives. Fasting is our best solution in helping to keep moving these filthy poisons out of our body!

Later in this book, we will explain how to examine your urine. After a few days of fasting, you will actually be able to see some of the poisons your body contained.

Medicine is only palliative. For behind disease lies the cause, and this cause no drug can reach. – Dr. Weir Mitchell

Rivers, Lakes, Oceans Becoming Polluted

Not only does the air we breathe fill our bodies with poisons, but our water is so filthy that more strong toxic chemicals are used to make it fit(?) to drink. An inorganic mineral called chlorine is used to supposedly help purify our drinking water . . . along with alum and many other inorganic minerals. Remember, your body can only absorb organic minerals from living plant matter. Any inorganic minerals must be eliminated from the body by the Vital Force. If it's below normal and can't keep up the cleansing, then these inorganic chemicals become lodged in the body's tissues to cause future problems!

Lake Erie is critically ill, and the symptoms are there for all to see. Beaches that once were gleaming with white sand are covered with odorous green slime. The lake's prize fish – walleye, blue pike, yellow perch, and whitefish – have all but disappeared. One Cleveland health student wrote to tell us that "Our lake is a wastebasket for factories. It is unfit for fish to live in, and for people to drink and use, because it's loaded with toxic, deadly chemicals." The major reason for the lake's terrible pollution is that most of its larger tributaries have been turned into little more than open sewers. Detroit alone pours 1.5 million gallons of waste a day into the Detroit River, which flows directly into Lake Erie.

The Cuyahoga River, which runs through the middle of Akron and Cleveland before spilling into the lake, is so clogged with logs, rotted pilings, chemicals, oil slicks and old tires that it has been labeled the filthiest water in America. Added to the scum and stench are thousands of dead fish that were smothered by the nasty pollution.

On a cruise up the Buffalo River last summer, Buffalo's mayor glided past islands of detergents, pools of grain dust and a general rainbow of dirty industrial discharge. "The odor was overpowering. Unbelievable! Disgusting!" he concluded. Hopefully, the Buffalo and Cuyahoga River environmental problems have now been corrected!

We are citing only one water supply among the many that are completely contaminated. All across America we find water supplies polluted. We use lots of water and it's so heavily chemicalized that it isn't fit to use.

Fasting – The Key to Internal Purification

Remember that all those inorganic chemicals must be passed out of your body or they can cause great damage. If the body's Vital Force drops too low then it can't force these inorganic chemicals through your eliminative systems. Then they remain in the body and can cause grave health damage in the future!

If we are to get these poisons out of our bodies we must fast. By fasting we give our bodies a physiological rest. This rest builds Vital Force. The more Vital Force we have, the more toxins are going to be eliminated from the body to help keep it clean, pure and healthy.

Poisons from Chemical Pesticides & Sprays

Tons upon tons of all varieties of deadly chemicals are not only sprayed in the air to kill insects, but many more tons are sprayed on commercially grown fruits and vegetables. Salads are healthy and appetizing, but often are made deadly because of the use of insecticide sprays. This year's crops have been exposed to more poisonous pesticide chemicals than ever before. You must be on guard and buy and eat organic produce for your health!

Beware of that salad! It may fill your body with deadly poisons! A convention group of women were having lunch at a Miami hotel and shortly afterwards, they were all seized with an attack of cramps. Nausea and dizziness soon followed. Sick, pale and shaken from vomiting, the women required medical aid. It didn't take a physician long to trace the source of this outbreak of acute poisoning. The villain proved to be an appetizing salad bar, consisting of vegetables, dressings, etc. Stating the reasons for the illness, the doctor said, "The poisoning was caused by chemicals, 'stay fresh' stabilizer spray and pesticides on restaurant's salad vegetables."

Dangerous chemical pesticides, insecticides and fertilizers are used on crops. Recently the FDA reported the seizure of endive and lettuce contaminated with excessive residues of toxic pesticide chemicals and parathion (a highly poisonous agricultural insecticide).

Food Crops Exposed to Toxic Poisons

Food shipments are often found exceeding the legal limits of toxic chemical pesticides and are seized. But this isn't the whole sad story of food poisoning. First of all, only shipments destined for interstate commerce are checked, and only a small fraction of the country's total produce ever comes under the scrutiny of an inspector. Many tons and truckloads of lettuce containing pesticide residues "in excess of legal tolerance" will stay within the state or community where they are grown and not be checked at all! As far as shipments across state lines, the U. S. Food and Drug Administration will be the first to admit that, because of limited manpower, only a fraction of the fruit and vegetable shipments in interstate commerce are checked.

The frightening truth is that a high percentage of the field crops you are eating have been sprayed with a wide variety of deadly poisons including chlorinated hydrocarbons, pesticides, herbicides, fungicides and other phosphorus and toxic compounds also used in growing such as toxic fertilizers. The contamination of salad vegetables doesn't stop with spraying the leafy portion of the plant. Medical researchers have discovered that many chemicals such as fertilizers and weed killers applied to the soil can remain there for a long time and are then absorbed by succeeding crops grown in the fields. The poison finally ends up in the pulp of the vegetable itself. It becomes part of it and cannot be washed off! Start demanding organic produce!

No doubt it has occurred to you that if the vegetables in your salad are contaminated you should make some effort to get rid of this poisonous residue before you eat too much of it. You might feel that peeling off the skin of a tomato or removing the outer layer of the lettuce will do the job. It won't. Some of the residue will be removed, certainly, but there will be more in lower leaves and in the pulp itself. The chemicals cannot even be broken down by cooking! The poison is part of the plant and is there to stay. So eat organic and don't panic!

Some students drink deeply at the fountain of knowledge – most only gargle.

Fasting Aids in Flushing
Deadly Poisons from the Body

When we fast (stop eating) all the Vital Force that has been used to convert food into energy and body tissue is now being used to flush poisons from the body! When Patricia and I travel throughout America and the world lecturing, we are fortunate to know health-minded people everywhere. We are usually well supplied with organically homegrown fruits and vegetables from their health gardens. But sometimes only commercially grown foods are available, which may have been sprayed with poisonous pesticides. But, we fast faithfully to cleanse toxins out, even when traveling, one 24 hour fast weekly.

I do four 7 to 10 day fasting periods yearly. When I go on a 7 to 10 day complete water fast, I take a specimen of my urine each morning upon arising. I put it in a small labeled bottle to let it cool and settle. In a few days, I can see little crystals forming in the urine. I have had my urine examined for chemicals, and the examiner has told me time and time again that traces of DDT and other deadly pesticide residues have appeared in my urine. On one occasion, I took a 21 day complete water fast. On the 19th day, I had terrible pains in my bladder. When I urinated it felt like red hot water passing through me. I had this urine examined and sure enough, it was filled with DDT and other poisons!

A great feeling of energy flowed over my body when this poison had passed out of it. The whites of my eyes were as clear as new snow. My body took on a pink glow and my energy surged. Now, remember I had been fasting for 19 days. Yet, I drove from Pasadena, California to Mt. Wilson, which is six thousand feet high, and climbed the trail with absolutely no fatigue! I ran with ease most of the way down the winding trail. I felt that a tremendous burden had been lifted from my body! In my personal opinion, fasting is the only way to rid the body of the many commercial poisons found in foods.

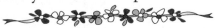

Who's Eating Fast Foods? Americans – 30 Billion Times a Year!
USA Today said 44% of junk food eaters are 35 years or older. Only 23% are youth under 17 years old. – Shocking Food Facts Causing Health Problems

Health Menace – Waxed Fruits & Vegetables!

Top medical experts reveal another menace to the nation's health – a toxic wax on fruits and vegetables. Next time you eat an apple, green pepper or cucumber, etc. take a good look at its surface. Is it bright, smooth and have a glossy look? If so, beware! Chances are it's coated with a wax paraffin solution which is one of America's most serious health threats, according to medical experts! Scratch surface to check for wax. The wax coating seals fruits and vegetables with a protective layer which they claim retains the water and juices, preserving the taste and creating a false appearance of freshness. It leaves a toxic wax residue that clogs the body!

What you are eating is a kind of wax that cannot be handled by your body – a paraffin wax which is a by-product of petroleum. There is no organ in your body, including the liver, that can process petroleum. This deadly wax therefore runs wild in the body. That is one reason doctors are so baffled by the many new diseases that American people are acquiring from eating foods contaminated by commercial food interests. Demand organic produce and unwaxed fruits and vegetables from all your produce markets - this helps get results!

This wax can cause damage if it remains in the body. If you keep eating waxed fruits and vegetables, the weekly 24 to 36 hour fast combined with the longer fasts during the year also helps in ridding your body of this deadly petroleum wax.

Fasting is a Miracle – I Thank Paul Bragg

I really haven't had any health problems since I was 17, when I started reading about health and nutrition, especially the Bragg Miracle of Fasting book. I started realizing there was a real connection between what you put in your mouth and your health and how you felt. So I immediately changed everything about my diet. I stopped eating refined white flour and sugar products, most dairy products and anything that was not a whole grain or whole food. What was left was a lot of healthy things: organic vegetables, fruits, legumes, seeds, nuts, etc. After years of asthma, within a month I could breath almost normally for the first time in my life. Fasting is a miracle and I thank Paul Bragg!

– Paul Wenner, Creator Gardenburger, author of *Garden Cuisine*

Food Supply Poisoned by Man

Thousands of synthetic food additives, chemicals, fertilizers and pesticides dumped into the nation's food and water supply are responsible for a great deal of sickness. For years our foods have been loaded with so-called "safe" chemicals that now have been discovered harmful to the human body. Sadly, many toxic pesticides are still being used! My friend, Rachel Carson, in her classic book, *Silent Spring*, exposed the harm the chemical industry was causing to the human population, as well as the environment and all wildlife. Please read *Silent Spring*, available at most libraries. It's a must read!

For example: take a loaf of commercially refined, "embalmed" white bread that's been treated, bleached, colored, dyed, enriched, purified, softened, preserved, flavored, and given a fresh odor – all by synthetic toxic chemicals that your body doesn't need or want!

In most stores it's almost impossible to get a healthy loaf of 100% whole grain bread that is free of toxic sprays and synthetic food additives. It's best to make your own bread or shop at health food stores for healthy whole grain products that are the real staff of life and health!

The amazing human body is a miraculous collection of individual cells. When nourished by healthy foods that provide the basic needs for growth and normal function, humans can live to 120 years or more! But when people toy with their body and pollute it with chemicalized, toxic, unhealthy foods, water and air, naturally the body responds adversely! When food is polluted and its entire composition altered by toxic chemicals, the body's cells become sick, function poorly and cannot keep adjusting to the irritating toxins forced on them – causing illness, premature ageing and death!

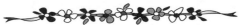

Wisdom is the principal thing; therefore get wisdom, and with all thy getting, get understanding. – Proverbs 4:7

It's not where we stand in the world, but in what direction we are moving.

Nothing can bring you peace but yourself. – Ralph Waldo Emerson

Synthetic, Toxic Food Additives Can Kill!

A vast amount of chemical poisons contaminate our food. Most commercial interests are not concerned with our health and lives. The economic bottom line is their main concern. It's best and safer to eat live, organically grown foods whenever possible. Avoid complicated, chemicalized, preserved foods. Read the labels of all foods you purchase! Ask questions about any special products and foods you like – even write the company and ask for a complete nutritional and chemical analysis.

Fast faithfully 24 – 36 hours weekly to rid yourself of toxins and help your body stay healthy and clean. When you don't feel up to par (colds, flus, mucus, pains, aches, etc.), then it's time to take a 3, 5 or 7 day complete fast and give your body a thorough body detox cleansing.

> **When you fast, your Vital Force is doing the cleansing.**

- If you are going to keep your body clean and healthy – you must fast faithfully!
- When you fast, wonderful miracles will happen in your body!
- The body is cleansing, repairing and healing itself!
- Follow a fasting regime of one day a week and you will feel greater than you have ever felt. Internal cleansing puts you on the road to Super Health.

Beware of Harmful Salt

Would you use sodium, a caustic alkali, to season your food? Or chlorine, a poisonous gas? "Ridiculous questions," you say. "Nobody would be foolhardy enough to do that." Of course not. But the shocking truth is that most people do just that because they don't know that these powerful chemicals constitute the inorganic crystalline compound known as salt. For centuries, the expression "salt of the earth" has been used to designate something good and essential. This idea is erroneous! Salt may actually help to bury you!

14

Happiness is not being pained in body or troubled in mind.
– Thomas Jefferson, 3rd U.S. President

Salt: Some Startling Facts:

- **Salt is not a food!** There is no more justification for its culinary use than there is for potassium chloride, calcium chloride, barium chloride or any other chemical on the druggist's shelf.

- **Salt cannot be digested, assimilated or utilized by the body.** Salt has no nutritional value! Salt has no vitamins, no organic minerals and no nutrients of any kind! Instead, it is harmful and causes trouble in the kidneys, bladder, heart, arteries, veins and blood vessels. Salt is the main cause of waterlogged tissues that cause swelling and edema (dropsy).

- **Salt may act as a heart poison.** It also can increase the irritability of the nervous system.

- **Salt acts to rob calcium from the body** and attacks the mucous lining throughout the body.

If salt is so dangerous to health, why is it used so widely? Mainly because it's a habit ingrained over the years. But it's a habit based on a serious misconception that the body needs it. But many people never eat salt and never miss it! Your wise body doesn't want it. Once a person is free of the salt habit, salt becomes repulsive to the taste as tobacco is to a nonsmoker! Among certain animal species, salt acts as a poison, particularly in the case of fowl. And pigs have been known to die after ingesting large doses of salt.

15

How Did the Salt Habit Originate?

Gustav von Bunge, a biochemist, explains that in prehistoric times there was a balance of organic sodium and potassium minerals in the earth. But continued rainfall over the centuries washed away the more soluble organic sodium salts. In time, many land-grown foods and soils became deficient in sodium, but high in potassium. The result was that animals and humans developed a craving for something to replace this mineral deficiency. They found an ineffective and highly dangerous substitute in salt (inorganic sodium chloride).

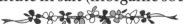

The Bragg Healthy Lifestyle followed daily will help you last a long lifetime!

Salt Causes Edema, Kidney Problems, etc.

Swallowing salt to obtain natural organic sodium is like taking inorganic calcium to get calcium. Both are chemicals and neither can be assimilated. All inorganic chemicals are harmful to the body, the digestive organs, etc. That's why the body sends out a sudden SOS thirst signal, a call for water, after salt is consumed! The stomach is reacting to salt and demands water to quickly flush the salt out through the kidneys. You can imagine what effect this has on the delicate kidney filters.

Millions suffer from kidney problems! Of all the body organs, the kidneys are most affected by salt. What happens when more salt is eaten than the kidneys can eliminate? The kidneys break down, the excess salt is deposited in various body parts, especially the lower extremities. To protect its tissues against salt, the body automatically seeks to dilute it by accumulating water in the needed areas to help flush out salt. As the tissues become waterlogged, swelling occurs in the feet, ankles and legs causing edema and dropsy. Salt also causes puffy eyelids and water bags below the eyes.

What Salt Does to Your Blood Pressure

Salt is harmful to the kidneys, and also injurious to the heart. In some heart conditions even a small amount can be dangerous! The action of the heart muscle is governed by the balance of natural, organic sodium and calcium salts in the blood. Salt tends to disturb this vital action, increasing the heartbeat and causing high blood pressure which affects millions!

Statistics show the Japanese have the highest blood pressure problems. What causes high blood pressure? Medical science recognizes many causes: salt, stress, toxic substances such as smoking and insecticide sprays, the side effects of drugs, food additives and toxic pollutants. To protect yourself from these caustic agents, exclude all the harmful agents possible from your environment. The major cause of high blood pressure you can definitely remedy: don't eat salt!

Are you in Health Bankruptcy? If so, you need a Health Overhaul!

Up to now, we have been talking about causing high blood pressure in the average person. But how about the effects of salt on those millions suffering from our country's most prevalent ailment, obesity? Here is a critical area for research, because excess weight is known to be frequently accompanied by high blood pressure. Is there a link between the overweight individual's high blood pressure and his salt intake? The answer is ahead!

The Myth of the "Salt Lick"

Is a low-salt diet a deficient diet? Don't we need plenty of salt in our diets to keep us in top physical condition? This is a popular notion, but is it true? People will tell you that animals will travel for miles to visit so called "salt licks". I investigated salt licks where wild forest animals congregate from miles around to lick the soil. Although all of these sites were known as "salt licks", the one chemical property they all had in common was a complete absence of sodium chloride. There was absolutely no organic or inorganic sodium at the salt licks. But they all had an abundance of other organic minerals and nutrients which the animals craved.

Why Cows are Given Large Amounts of Salt

A man who puts his investment in a dairy farm is in it to make all the profit he can. Dairy farmers have found that by giving cows salt blocks to lick, they drink more water. The more water they drink, the more milk they produce. Most cows are sick, mass fed and drugged.

But the result is that the average quart of milk contains the extremely high content of 1½ grams (1,500 mgs) of salt per quart! Go past any American school and look at the children. You will be amazed by how many of them are overweight, lack stamina and the spark of youth. Most are heavy drinkers of commercial milk, and most foods they eat contain high concentrations of salt.

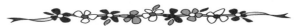

The best way to lengthen life is to avoid shortening it.

It's strange that some men will drink and eat anything put before them, but check very carefully the oil put in their car.

Americans Are Salt-a-holics!

Go into supermarkets and look at canned, bottled and frozen foods. All of them are loaded with salt! Plus there's salt in milk, ice cream, prepared vegetables and most commercial foods. Add it all up and you can see why heart disease is the # 1 killer in America! We are a nation of salt-a-holics! Cheese, frozen and canned vegetables, breads, potato and corn chips, and most all popular foods are saturated with salt. Even commercial baby foods contain salt! Read labels! Don't buy salt!

Death Valley Hike Proved Salt Dangerous

Most people have the preconceived idea that salt lost through perspiring must be immediately replaced. Many factories supply salt tablets to their workers. They mistakenly believe these are helpful! But are these salt tablets necessary? In my opinion: "NO!"

To prove definitely to myself that I did not need salt during extremely hot weather, I went to Death Valley, California, one of the hottest spots in the entire world during July and August. On my first test I hired 10 husky young college athletes to make the hike in Death Valley from Furnace Creek Ranch to Stovepipe Wells, a distance of approximately 30 miles.

The boys had salt tablets and all the water they could drink . . . and a station wagon filled with plenty of food that contained salty foods like bread, buns, crackers, cheese, luncheon meats and hot dogs. They each ate, drank and took as many salt tablets as they desired. I had no salt and I fasted during the 30 mile hike. We began the hike on a sweltering July morning. The higher the sun rose, the hotter it became! Up went the heat until at noon it stood at 130 degrees – a dry, hot heat that seemed to want to melt and defeat us!

18

Water is the essential fluid of life . . . the solvent of our ills and the deliverer of a radiant long life.

Use your willpower and better judgement to select and eat only the foods which are best for you, regardless of the ridicule or gibes of your friends or acquaintances. – Dr. Richard T. Field

The college boys gobbled the salt tablets and guzzled quarts of cool water. For lunch they drank cola drinks with ham and cheese sandwiches. We rested a half hour after lunch and then continued our rugged hike across the red hot blazing sands. Soon things were beginning to happen to those strong, husky college boys.

First, 3 of them got violently ill and threw up all they had eaten and drunk for lunch. They got dizzy and turned deathly pale and great weakness overcame them. They quit the hike immediately! They were driven back to the Furnace Creek Ranch in poor condition. But the hike went on with 7 college athletes continuing. As we hiked, they drank large amounts of cold water and took more salt tablets. Then suddenly 5 of them got stomach cramps and became deathly ill. Up came the water and their lunch. These 5 had to be driven back to the ranch.

That left but 2 out of 10 hikers. It was now about 4 pm and the merciless sun beat down on us with great fury. Almost on the hour, the last remaining salt tablet-eating athlete collapsed under that hot, burning sun and had to be rushed back to the ranch for medical care.

Only the Non-Salt User Finishes Hike

That left me alone on the test . . . and I felt as fresh as a daisy! I was not full of salt tablets and I was not full of food because I was on a complete fast. The college boys wanted cold water, but I drank only pure distilled water, not chilled. I finished the 30 mile hike in around 10½ hours and I had no ill effects whatsoever! I camped out for the night. The next day I arose and hiked another 30 miles back to the ranch without food or salt tablets.

The doctors gave me a thorough examination and found me in perfect condition. I am ready and willing to repeat this hike across Death Valley, California for any scientific group that wants to do research on man's mythical "need" for salt.

Mother Nature is man's teacher. She unfolds her treasures to his search, unseals his eyes, illuminates his mind and purifies his heart. – Alfred B. Street

Change your mind and change to a healthy lifestyle and your life and body will sparkle with health and joy! – Patricia Bragg

Historical Proof Salt is Not Needed

Rommel's German-Afrikan Corps swept across the gates of Egypt, fought and lost a hard battle at El Alamein. Then they retreated over miles of blazing desert. Yet, when the war was over, the English found the captured troops in good physical condition, even though the German soldiers were not supplied with salt tablets. This story – just as my own Death Valley hike, which was also performed in the blazing desert sun – supports the findings of many experiments performed on humans with a non-salt diet under hot desert conditions.

What happens, according to the scientific studies, is that: after the first few days of becoming acclimatized, the subjects stop losing salt through perspiration. Apparently there is a normalizing mechanism at work that conserves the sodium in the body. The comfortable endurance during all weather conditions of people on rigid, salt-poor diets shows that the "need" for added salt in hot weather has been greatly exaggerated.

There is enough naturally occurring sodium in vegetables, celery, soy beans, seaweeds and other foods that have not been processed or supplemented with common table salt. These natural foods can supply the needed organic sodium required by the body. Proof of this is also found in the past histories of many races throughout the world who have never used salt.

The Native Americans knew nothing about salt when the first explorers landed. Columbus and all the explorers of the American continent found wonderful physical specimens when they arrived. Sad fact – the physical degeneration of people often follows the introduction of salt, alcohol, refined foods and toxic chemicals.

I have made over 13 expeditions to the far corners of the earth and I never found the inhabitants to be salt users. Therefore, none of them suffered from high blood pressure. In fact, regardless of age, they generally had blood pressures of 120 over 80, which is perfect. They did not suffer from kidney or heart diseases, either.

Ruts long traveled grow comfortable.

How Much Salt Can the Body Tolerate Daily?

There's been a great deal of research on salt tolerance. The American Heart Association recommends that healthy adults reduce their sodium intake to no more than 2400 milligrams per day. But the body's actual physiological sodium requirement is less than 500 mg daily. The average American salt addict actually consumes 2 to 5 times his sodium tolerance daily!

This extremely high salt figure Americans eat is due to the excessive amount of "hidden salt" in almost all commercially prepared foods. It's in breads, cheese, prepared meats (ham, bacon, lunch meats, etc.), frozen and canned veggies, soups and hundreds of staple foods.

I was born and reared in Virginia and many of my relatives suffered from high blood pressure. They died early of strokes and kidney diseases because they were heavy salt, pork, ham, sausage and bacon eaters. High concentrations of table salt were used at every meal. By the time these people were 30 years old, they ached all over with what they called the "misery." Their joints were cemented, and they hobbled around stiffly and with great pain! I believe that the heavy salt diet of the average Southerner brought on this "misery."

The most dramatic wrongful death case against salt occurred in a Binghamton, New York hospital, where a number of babies died when salt was inadvertently used in their formula. An overdose of salt can kill a baby quickly. The body needs natural, organic sodium – not table salt, an inorganic chemical. You can obtain natural sodium which Mother Nature provides in organic form in celery, beets, carrots, potatoes, soybeans, turnips, sea vegetation, seaweed, kelp, watercress, etc. and many other natural, healthy foods. Remember, only organic minerals can be utilized by your body's living cells.

It's magnificent to live long if one keeps healthy and youthful. – Harry Fosdick

I have found that distilled water is a sovereign remedy for my rheumatism. I attribute my almost perfect health largely to distilled water. – Dr. Alexander Graham Bell, *Telephone Inventor*

Fasting De-Salts Body Cells and Organs

I have had over 70 years experience with the science and use of rational fasting. And I have found that in 4 days of complete fasting we can de-salt the body. The urine will reveal the story of salt. Take a 4 day complete distilled water fast. Nothing must pass through your body for 4 days, except for distilled water and ACV drink. Drink at least 8 to 10 glasses daily to flush the salt out.

Each morning take a sample of the first urine your body passes. Put these urine bottles (labeled) on a shelf to settle for 3 weeks, then look at them in the sunlight. You will see concentrated salt and toxic wastes in the bottom of the bottle. When this salt is passed from your body notice how freely your kidneys will function. Notice how naturally moist your mouth is and how you have no abnormal thirst. Notice your skin and muscle tone. The first thing the body throws off during a fast is salt and the side effects – bloating and edema (dropsy) that goes with salt. Lumpy, waterlogged spots vanish and you become more streamlined. There is a thinner and more youthful look to your body. Water-bloating vanishes and you begin to see your natural figure again.

You can hardly believe your eyes. A wonderful transformation is taking place during your fast. The powerful Vital Force that would otherwise be used to handle your food is now being used exclusively to clean out the debris, waste, and poisons that have been locked in the body cells and vital organs. Rejuvenation is taking place in every one of the billions of cells of the body! After the 4 days of de-salting the body, be sure to keep salt out of your diet. It's a difficult thing to do since there's so much "hidden salt" in so many different foods. That is where your weekly 24 to 36 hour fast helps to continue to de-salt your body.

We find it difficult in our world travels, lecturing and doing research, to avoid "hidden salt" in foods, even though we always request, "No salt, please!" in restaurants, on cruise ships, airplanes and trains. However, our weekly cleansing fast of 24 to 36 hours keeps any inorganic salt we ate flowing out of our bodies.

We never add salt to foods in the Bragg household! We use natural seasonings that add zest to foods: herbs, garlic, onion, lemon and our delicious Bragg Apple Cider Vinegar and Bragg Liquid Aminos, a tasty all purpose soy seasoning that contains 16 amino acids. With fasting, you'll soon see how much better you feel and look! And what a sweet taste you will have in your mouth. You will note many other changes for the better when you are faithful with your fasting program and banish salt.

Fasting is the Great Cleanser and Purifier

People are constantly asking and writing me, "Will a fast cure my 'this or that' disease?" I want it clearly and distinctly understood that I am not recommending fasting as a cure for any disease! I don't believe in cures unless Mother Nature, God and your body do it! I can only inspire you to fast to build more Vital Force to overcome enervation and debilitation. Then as you build up your body's Vital Force it can then self-cleanse and self-heal. Read our *Build Powerful Nerve Force* book for more info on Vital Force.

23

Enervation Explained

We live in a chaotic world. The demands for energy in these hectic times are enormous. We all have a standard of living to maintain and an image to create and live up to for our relatives and friends. We each have many responsibilities. Every waking hour requires great outputs of Vital Force to earn our daily living, to support our family, to drive a car in traffic, to be responsible for a job, to maintain a house, to rear our children, to perform social and civic duties. Plus there are thousands of other daily activities that call for your Vital Force to perform continually in operating your body. You need go-power and energy!

Energy is a precious ingredient; it cannot be purchased in a bottle or can. Many misguided people think they can get it from drugs, alcohol, tobacco, caffeine, sugar and colas. They can't! Energy is a reward for living as close to Mother Nature's Laws as possible.

Humans Won't Take Blame for Miseries

It's because of your bad habits that things start to break down and decay in your body! Your bad habits enervate and rob your energy! This is the important point: as energy drops and you become enervated, you do not have enough energy for your body to properly cleanse. Low energy brings on slow functioning in all the basic eliminative organs: the bowels, kidneys, skin and lungs. There is no energy to function at full natural capacity. Then poisons of all kinds are not completely flushed out of the body, but instead are deposited inside, slowly building up and taking a terrible toll!

Poisons start to collect in various parts of the body, causing you illness, aches and pains. These are Mother Nature's flashing warning signals that you are not living the healthy lifestyle that She and God intended for your body! Perhaps you blame everything and everybody for your problems, instead of analyzing your lifestyle habits for the real causes!

"No," you say, "I caught a cold when I worked too hard." "I get sick because I am getting older." Excuse after excuse is given . . . but never the real cause: yourself. You alone are responsible for your aches, pains and premature ageing! Start now living The Bragg Healthy Lifestyle!

Your unhealthy habits promote low Vital Force and fatigue! Then the poisons can't be thoroughly flushed out of the body. So they find a spot to torment you and are named according to the location of your pain. But that pain actually came from the way you live. Don't put the blame elsewhere! You have enervated yourself, and the toxic poisons from many sources of your daily living are tormenting you. Cleanse and rebuild your Vital Force by fasting and natural living, and fatigue will vanish! Unhealthy living is the reason why you feel burned out, fatigued, full of aches and pains, prematurely old and, maybe heading straight for the human "scrap heap"!

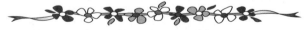

*When you live as God and Mother Nature
intended you to live, you start to rejuvenate yourself!*

Most people think they can attempt to break all of Mother Nature's good and just laws of Healthful Living. How very wrong they are. You can never break a natural law – it will break you! Many think they can break all of the natural laws of health – then run to a doctor to circumvent these natural laws by having a medical "miracle" fix-all bandage for their misery.

The Miracles Are Within You

The human being craves sudden miracles. Not fully aware of the actual achievements of natural nutrition, exercise and fasting – which are in themselves miraculous – he searches in the realm of the unknown for manifestations that he cannot understand. Simply obeying Mother Nature's great laws is too simple a procedure to follow! People full of miseries and premature ageing want a quick, easy way to find health and youthfulness. Just remember: You must earn your health! You cannot buy it. No one can give it to you. I have boundless energy, great power, wonderful strength and radiant, vibrant health because I have studied with respect Mother Nature and God's Natural Laws and followed them faithfully! These healthy, natural nutritional laws, the Laws of Self-Purification – fasting, keeping the circulation healthy, free-flowing and the skin and muscle tone active by exercise – lead to agelessness.

Do You Have Harmful Habits to Overcome?

Do you eat salt and salty foods? Do you drink coffee? Use tobacco? Alcohol? Use refined white sugar or eat products with this devitalized material in it? What devitaminized and demineralized foods are dragging you down and enervating you? Is your willpower weak or strong? Who is the boss of your body? Your bad habits? Or does your mind control your appetites? Remember that flesh is dumb and can't think for you. Only with positive thinking can you overcome the bad habits that your flesh might crave. If you really crave glorious health, unbelievable strength, tremendous vital force and a trim and fit body you will be proud of, start working with Mother Nature today and not against her!

Fasting – the Key to Super Energy

Fasting is the key which unlocks Mother Nature's storehouse of energy. It reaches every cell in the body, the inner organs and generates the Life Forces. No one can do it for you! It's a personal duty that only you can perform. No one can eat for you. And I believe that 99% of all human suffering is caused by wrong and unnatural eating. The efficiency of any machine depends upon the quality and amount of fuel for generating power it is given. And that goes double for the human machine!

Some people will blame everything on earth except food as the cause of their physical miseries and premature ageing. Why they are suffering is always a mystery to them. The average person does not know how horribly unclean the inside of their body is, caused by years and years of overeating, eating when not really hungry and, in many cases, wrong-minded eating of dead, devitalized foods. All these unhealthy habits build up internal poisons and clogging toxic wastes in their bodies.

Put the person who brags that he "enjoys perfect health" on a complete distilled water fast for 5 or 6 days. His breath will become putrid and his tongue will have a foul-smelling, white coating. His urine will become dark and evil-smelling. This definitely proves that his whole body is filled up with decayed and uneliminated toxic materials brought in by eating the wrong foods.

The continual accumulation of increasingly foul body poison is the buried or latent unknown ailment. When Mother Nature wants to get rid of this ailment by a "crisis" commonly known as sickness, people look for an easy "quick fix" to get rid of their troubles. They usually ignore the miraculous one Mother Nature has given us which has no dangerous side effects: FASTING!

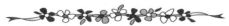

Now learn what and how great benefits a temperate diet will bring along with it. In the first place, you will enjoy good health. – Horace, 65 B.C.

Over the next decade nutritionists expect to see those pursuing the more healthy lifestyle move from meat to beans to avoid saturated fat, toxins and cholesterol found in all animal products. – Reader's Digest

Fasting – A Natural Instinct and Great Purifier

Sickness is Mother Nature's way of showing you that you are filled with toxic wastes and internal poison. Dead people don't have colds. It is only when you are alive and have Vital Force that you have physical problems. By fasting, you are working with Mother Nature to help expel the wastes and poisons you have accumulated in your body. Every animal in the wilderness knows fasting, for it's the only method animals use to help overcome any physical trouble that befalls them. This is pure animal instinct. We humans have lived so long in this soft civilization that we have lost this natural instinct to fast when health problems occur in our bodies.

In your life you may have experienced physical suffering, when you felt no desire for food – it might even have repulsed you. Then, kind but ignorant relatives or friends may have told you to "eat to keep up your strength." The very last thing you needed was food, because your body was signaling you to stop eating. Mother Nature wanted you to fast so she could use your Vital Force to cleanse and then heal your body.

The soft voice of Mother Nature is often hard to hear and understand. By fasting, your extra-sensory instinct becomes very keen. The fast sharpens your mind and tunes you in with the gentle inner voice of Mother Nature and God. Fasting has made my inner body, mind and soul alert! My body and mind work better after each fast. I know yours will, too! Fasting is for sure a miracle!

Fasting clears away the thousand little things which quickly accumulate and clutter the body, mind and heart. It cuts through corrosion and renews our contract with God and Mother Earth.

When health is absent, wisdom cannot reveal itself, strength cannot be exerted, wealth is useless and reason is powerless. – Herophiles, 300 B.C.

Fasting Saves You 15% Yearly Off Your Food Bill

Do you want to live a longer, happier, healthier life and save hundreds of dollars annually? Following The Bragg Healthy Lifestyle with water fasting one day a week not only provides life extension values, but an extra big savings of 15% off your annual food bill. – Patricia Bragg

Jesus, His Disciples and
Many Great Teachers Fasted

When the great city of Alexandria, Egypt was the educational center of the world, people had to fast for 40 days before they could enter and study with the master of that time. Jesus fasted for 40 days, and his disciples also took long fasts. All of history's great spiritual teachers have had great confidence in the power of fasting – not only to improve the physical body, but to promote a keener spiritual understanding of the divine power that is above us and within us. Your mental power increases! Prove it to yourself. See how much sharper and more alert your mind becomes after a fast. Notice how quickly you acquire facts . . . how much more your mind absorbs and remembers what you read.

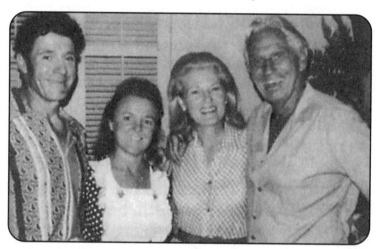

Jack LaLanne, Patricia Bragg, Elaine LaLanne & Paul C. Bragg
Jack says, "Bragg saved my life at age 15 when I attended the Bragg Health Crusade in Oakland, California." From that day, Jack has continued to live The Bragg Healthy Lifestyle and inspire millions to health and fitness.

Fasting is Cleansing, Purifying and Restful. – Meir Schneider

Jesus lived by His own rules. He fasted. – Matthew 6:16

When thou fastest appear not unto men to fast, but unto thy Father which is in secret: and thy Father, which seeth in secret, shall award thee openly. – Matthew 6:17-18

Chapter 3

The Enemy Within Our Bodies

Victor Hugo eloquently called the poison in our body "the serpent which is in man." While this remark is poetic, it contains even more truth than poetry. I have come to regard autointoxication (self-poisoning) as the worst enemy in the fight for Agelessness and Longevity. It is mind-poisoning as well as body-poisoning because, even after the energy of the body is regained, one has a lingering sense of the futility of all endeavors. Some are inclined to say, "The best of life is behind me. What lies before is brief and burdensome. So many of my friends and relations have gone." Others say, "My turn's coming. I've got a date with the undertaker and it's not so far off." These depressing thoughts generate sad moods and are detrimental to Agelessness and Longevity. Remember, you can make the second half of life the best.

29

Autointoxication itself is your health's greatest enemy. It's so common and yet so rarely recognized. Those morbid moods – the worry, tensions, stresses, frustrations, nervousness and needless anxiety – are foreign to a healthy state. You should always be optimistic, happy, carefree, self-confident and at peace. Why is it that sometimes when fortune smiles her brightest, you remain unhappy, mirthless, depressed, and ungrateful? Then again when things look their bleakest, you are amazed at your buoyancy. The purity or impurity of your bloodstream might explain that!

I love life and want to live 120 years and more in prime physical condition! Each day of life is a beautiful, priceless miracle. I want to keep it, value it, treasure it and enjoy every waking hour! I also want this for you.

Money will buy a bed, but not sleep; books, but not brains; food, but not appetite; finery, but not beauty; a house, but not a home; medicine, but not health; luxuries, but not culture; amusements, but not happiness; religion, but not salvation.

Rid Yourself of Depression

The worst aspect of autointoxication is that it has been building up for years. It takes water fasting, whole natural foods and living a healthy lifestyle to defeat it. When these poisons are surging through your body, you often are pessimistic with depressed feelings. The mockery of life comes home to you. You begin to wonder, "Is it all worthwhile?" Then one morning you awaken to find your cheery self again. Though a bit shaken up, you have hopefully beaten off the foe. Newspapers, magazines, TV and radio all sell products that make promises to relieve you of that "half alive" feeling. Which one do you take? There are no shortcuts to feeling your best physically and mentally and looking your best.

You are punished by your bad habits of living!
You are greatly rewarded by your good habits of living!

Old Mother Nature will not let you get away with abusing your body. You must pay a high price every time you insult your body with dead and devitalized foods. Of course, you could take drugs to deaden or stimulate your body, but you are living in a fool's paradise if you think you can eat any old thing and then swallow some kind of magic pill and get away with it. You pay a dear price every time you make a garbage can of your stomach! Your heart and arteries suffer. Your spells of autointoxication (self-poisoning) are shortening your life. Each attack leaves its mark and, for this reason, it's something to dread. Please don't poison your bloodstream. Learn to defend and protect yourself against all possible autointoxication by living The Bragg Healthy Lifestyle.

Once a week make it a habit to take a complete water fast, lasting from 24 to 36 hours. On the days you do eat, consume only natural, organic and unpoisoned foods. Let your mind rule your body. Flesh is dumb! You can feed your stomach anything. Now you are going to use common sense and eat with new health intelligence.

The nervous system falters and suffers when we don't take care of our body.

Unhealthy Lifestyle & Overeating are Killers

Keep this firmly in mind: autointoxication is the greatest enemy of vibrant health. It's the root cause of all major physical troubles, because illness starts in a poisoned bloodstream. It's the basis of most troubles which affect the heart, arteries, liver, kidneys and joints. When your bloodstream, your river of life, becomes poisoned, this has more to do with premature ageing than all other causes combined. Keeping your blood pure, clean and healthy is half the battle! The other killer is overloading your stomach and digestive system, giving it a new job before it has finished digesting the previous meal.

You have been taught to eat at regular times, even if not hungry. Many, when it's mealtime, stuff themselves automatically. This is wrong and scientifically outdated, for overstuffing your body is very unhealthy!

Patricia and I took a cruise around South America visiting 12 countries. The over-stuffed passengers started with an early wake-up breakfast in their staterooms. Then an hour or so later they ate in the dining room a formal breakfast of bacon, ham, eggs, rolls, toast, jam, fried potatoes and gallons of coffee, followed by snacks on deck at mid-morning. Then a big buffet lunch at noon, afternoon tea with gooey pastries at 4 pm, a big supper at 7 pm and another big buffet at 11 pm. We buried 5 people at sea in a few short weeks! All died by autointoxications! This kind of overeating encourages fermentation, putrefaction, illness and death!

Life is a Slow Suicide For Many

From the cradle many begin damaging their health while lightheartedly trimming off the years quickly at the beginning of existence, unknowingly chopping them off in bigger chunks at the end. Blissfully unconscious, they burn their candles at both ends and sometimes even in the middle! Many people suffer in poor health not realizing that their unhealthy lifestyle habits are the main cause of their sickness.

To lengthen thy life, lessen thy meals. – Ben Franklin

Why Not Enjoy Life to 120?

There is little doubt that any person born with a sound constitution, according to health research and Genesis 6:3, can reach the 120 year mark! Why not? There are no diseases of old age. Now, follow me: if starting from childhood, you eat healthy, plus fast one day a week and several times a year for periods of from 7 to 10 days – then how is it possible to get a fatal disease?

Children today are being fed wrong! Many mothers don't nurse their babies. Some lack the internal vitality to produce the greatest food in the world for their young - mothers' milk. Their babies are bottle-fed and are given processed baby food out of jars, all loaded with refined white flours, sugar and dangerously full of deadly salt. The abuse of the physical machine of the modern child is started at birth. Under these tragic circumstances, sooner or later premature breakdown is inevitable.

If you seek enlightenment on the subject of health, look at people around you. Every day, there are 25 million Americans critically ill in thousands of hospitals from coast to coast. Three hundred thousand doctors are kept frantically busy trying to patch up the desperately sick people in our country! Over one hundred fifty thousand dentists can't do even 10% of the dental work Americans need! Avoid toxic silver fillings, fluoride water, toothpastes, gels, etc. Read the Bragg book *Water – The Shocking Truth*.

I find most children's mouths are filled with decay and cavities before they are 17. We are a desperately sick, ill nation! We are brainwashed to believe we are a healthy and vital country. But the facts and figures tell a different story. Even if you don't overeat, the food you eat is mostly unhealthy. Yet a little knowledge of physiology, health, diet and fasting could save you from health bankruptcy. Ignorance is a worse enemy than over indulgence. Overhaul your body and save your precious health! You can't be a walking toxic factory and expect to live a long life of super health in a painless, tireless, ageless body.

Man's days shall be 120 years. – Genesis 6:3

Autointoxication Promotes Sickness

I was reared in Virginia on a typical southern diet. Ninety percent of my food was prepared in the frying pan: fried chicken, fried ham, bacon, potatoes, pork chops and other fried meats of all kinds. I ate heavy cream, flour gravies and hot biscuits and plenty of pies, cakes and jellies. When I look back, I see I suffered in my youth from this self-poisoning and didn't know it. Despite my abhorrence of drugs, I let myself be drugged by the poisons within me. Rarely was I entirely free of them, and the average health I enjoyed was far from the radiant health that was my natural heritage.

I usually slept 10 hours a night instead of 8, and the excess I am sure was largely due to autointoxication. Even after a long night of sleep, I seldom woke up feeling refreshed, plus I had a bitter morning taste in my mouth.

Most people are not really living; they are merely existing. They are so full of toxic poisons that living becomes an effort. Few people rise early to see the sunrise and greet the new day with eagerness and joy! I do now!

Let us look at our bedrooms as recharge areas where we are required to spend a certain length of time in sleep to recharge our life batteries. Let's make our bedrooms uncluttered and peaceful with ample fresh air and light. Ceiling fans in hot summers are nice. During the early morning hours you always get more accomplished – so try to cultivate early morning rising. You can if you put your mind to it! Work days, when you get up earlier, take a "cat nap" for 20 minutes after eating your lunch.

I understand why millions worldwide use stimulants such as tobacco, alcohol, coffee, tea, cola drinks and "pep pills." They try to fight the desperate moods of fatigue and depression caused by autointoxication. I could write pages depicting the woes of toxins. As a youth my blood was poisoned. No one would set out to foul their pure bloodstream, yet, consistently, in ignorance I polluted my precious life with unhealthy foods. Analyze your life and improve where needed.

Outwit Acidosis That Affects Millions

It has taken me all these years of research and study to discover the great fact that the bloodstream should be alkaline. Yet, with most of us, it is in an acid state. From headache and indigestion, to pimples and the common cold, most problems arise from acidosis due to self-poisons caused by unhealthy foods. When the life stream is so polluted, how can our immune system defend the body against disease and illness? People unwittingly prepare the body for sickness with their unhealthy lifestyle and then let it be out of control, while they search for a magic pill that will work miracles!

Now if you are as naive as I was, you will ask, "What can I do to counteract this supposed acidity? How can I cleanse my blood?" The answer is: "By supplying it with alkaline-forming healthy foods." At the first sign of acidosis (heartburn, bloating, tired, etc.) go on a 3 day water fast. After fasting, switch to alkaline-forming healthy foods and be wise, always avoid unhealthy foods!

What Are Alkaline-Forming Foods?

"But what are alkaline-forming foods?" You ask. They are, generally speaking, organic, raw fruits and vegetables, salads and leafy greens and lightly steamed vegetables. Three-fifths of your diet should be composed of fruits and vegetables, both raw and cooked. It's always best to enjoy your raw fresh fruit or a raw vegetable garden salad before you eat any cooked foods. See recipe on page 231.

The alkaline forming foods are the most important to your body. Some of you will say, "raw fruits and vegetables give me gas, etc." That is because you are on the acid side and, when you eat the alkaline foods, they start to houseclean and move the toxins out of your bloodstream and body. So you avoid eating them and use the weak excuse that they don't agree with you. They do agree with you and your toxic body definitely needs them to help get you clean, healthy and alkaline!

Stop your life from an out-of-control spiral! Become the Health Captain of your life by following The Bragg Healthy lifestyle – start today!

Raw, Organic Fruits and Vegetables
Are Mother Nature's Miracle Cleansers

When you get a bad reaction from certain raw fruits and vegetables, remember that these are cleansing and purifying foods. Use a small amount until you can reduce your body's toxic poisons. Your weekly 24 hour fast is going to get rid of a lot of your body wastes. If you have the intestinal strength to fast for 3 to 7 days, most troubles from cleansing foods disagreeing with you will be over. What are the acid-forming foods? Chiefly sugar, its products and coffee, tea, alcohol, meats and fish.

No doubt the idea of excluding even a portion of the latter will dismay you, but if you want to live agelessly you must do many things at first that dismay you. Eventually you will be dismayed at your dismay. Often a new task is difficult because you think it will be. Tackle it with the idea that it is easy and it becomes easier! Living on a diet composed mainly of organic fruits, veggies, salads, nuts and seeds isn't difficult. No one will deny that fruits are luscious. Salads may be enjoyed in great variety. The list of vegetables is long and diversified. All the raw nuts and seeds, raw or lightly roasted pecans, almonds, walnuts, sunflower seeds, sesame seeds, etc. are nutritious and delicious. You need not confine yourself to these foods, but if you lean towards acidosis you should combine fasting with a diet of fruits, salads and veggies.

If you must eat meat, it should be only 2 or 3 times weekly. On the least symptom of feeling bad, get back to the healthier vegetarian alkaline diet quickly. Headaches, dizziness, specks in the vision, bitterness in the mouth, body fatigue and mental blockage merely denote a bile attack, but again the disorder may be more deep seated. If you think it's your liver, you should cut out all fats and flesh foods. Also, cut out all refined sugars and refined starches. The little protein you need you can get from organic healthy plant sources, beans, raw nuts and seeds, etc. The Vegetable Protein % Chart on page 233 will give you some healthy ideas.

Bad cooking dimishes happiness and shortens life. – Wisdom of Ages

Your Mind Must Control Your Body

Prudently assume, that your condition is one of autointoxication. If you feel your energy is at a low ebb, and not up to par, go on a short fast lasting from 24 hours to 3 or 4 days. Drink nothing but pure, steam distilled water. I will tell you more about water later.

You will experience a craving for food. But not an actual hunger. It's the body reflexes that are accustomed to being fed at certain intervals. Again let me state, *"Flesh is dumb!"* It has all kinds of cravings, but you must be its master. You must control your entire body with your mind. I can readily admit that fasting takes immense determination and willpower.

I remember very well my first 4 day fast. It was while I was under the care of the famous Dr. A. Rollier at his Switzerland sanitarium. I was battling for my life with tuberculosis and I had been at the sanitarium for several months. Dr. Rollier told me it was going to be a great experience – and it surely was! The good doctor told me to study my urine daily. So each day I took a specimen of my urine and kept it in a bottle. I put it on a shelf in my room and I would look at the specimens each day. As the urine would cool and settle I could see the great amount of foreign matter that was leaving my body.

As soon as I finished the fast, I was placed on a highly alkaline diet with an abundance of fresh fruits and raw and lightly steamed or baked vegetables. About 2 weeks after the fast, I experienced a sense of exhilaration and well-being that I had never known in my entire life.

From that time on my health and vitality grew by leaps and bounds. That was not my only fast under Dr. Rollier's supervision. He started me out with a 24 hour weekly fast and in the next 9 months, put me on a 7, 14 and 21 day fast. Between fasts I was fed an alkaline diet.

We live not upon what we eat, but upon what we digest. – Abernethy

It's never too late to begin getting into shape, but it does take daily perseverance. – Thomas K. Cureton

When it comes to health, nine men in ten are suicides. – Ben Franklin

Keep Your Stomach Healthy & Alkaline

Because acidosis is more of a negative than a positive ill, you should beware of it. Have you ever said, "Oh, I'm a little off color; low on energy; a bit blue for no real reason. Everyone has their off days. It seems to be a part of life." Nothing of the kind! You can maintain yourself in a state of consistent good health, not spasmodic good health. You can come to consider your body a fine machine, one that with proper care will never go wrong.

At the first suspicion of acidosis, analyze your diet. A grayish tongue, a snappish temper, a flushing of the face; these are not too trivial to heed! They are signs of danger! Perhaps today they might not amount to much, but tomorrow they will be more insistent. Acidosis is insidious and accumulative in its action; and it is today, not tomorrow, that you should begin to defend yourself, for life is self-defense. Your adversary has you at a disadvantage, and what you lack in stamina you must make up for in living a healthy lifestyle!

Beware then of acidosis and all of the evils it invites. Apart from asking for trouble from invading germs, chronic acidosis will lead to high blood pressure and followed by arteriosclerosis (hardening of the arteries). Thus, the chain is completed: over-acid dietary autointoxication, high blood pressure, stiff arteries and then premature death. High-sugar, high-fat and high-protein diets promote acidosis. Stay away from them! Eat a healthy diet rich in fruits, vegetables and grains from organic sources. At the first danger sign, be strong and give up all unhealthy habits and faithfully live The Bragg Healthy Lifestyle. This will guide you to super health!

When you live The Bragg Healthy Lifestyle you can help activate your own powerful internal defense arsenal and maintain it at top efficiency. However, bad, unhealthy eating habits make it harder for your body to fight off illness! – Paul C. Bragg

What wound did ever heal but by gentle degrees. – William Shakespeare

Little things are like weeds – the longer we neglect them the larger they grow.

Perfect Balancer – Apple Cider Vinegar

Another safeguard to keep your acid/alkaline balance healthy is to enjoy the healthy Bragg Organic Raw Apple Cider Vinegar Cocktail three times daily. Drink a glass upon arising, another an hour before lunch and one an hour before dinner. The mixture is 1 to 2 tsp. each of Bragg ACV and raw honey in a glass of distilled water.

Important Parts of the Digestive System

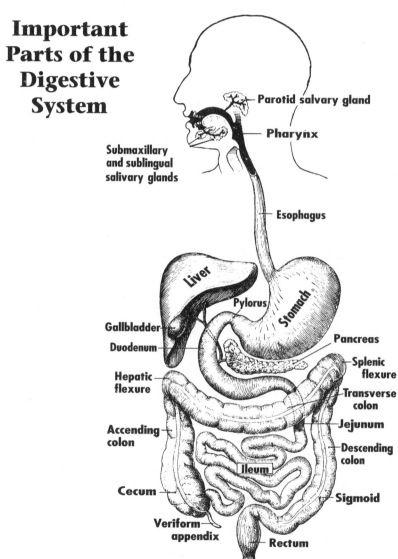

- Parotid salvary gland
- Pharynx
- Submaxillary and sublingual salivary glands
- Esophagus
- Liver
- Pylorus
- Stomach
- Gallbladder
- Pancreas
- Duodenum
- Splenic flexure
- Hepatic flexure
- Transverse colon
- Accending colon
- Jejunum
- Descending colon
- Ileum
- Cecum
- Sigmoid
- Veriform appendix
- Rectum

Organic Raw Unfiltered Apple Cider Vinegar with the "Mother" is the #1 food I recommend for maintaining the body's vital acid-alkaline balance.
– Gabriel Cousens, M.D., Author of *"Conscious Eating"*

Chapter 4

Fasting Fights Deadly Acid Crystals

Toxic Acid Crystals Can Cement Your Joints to Make You Stiff

Stand on any street corner and watch the average person hobble along. Their feet, knees, hips, spine and head seem to be cemented. There is no free-swinging movement in their locomotion. Let's look at their feet. They seem to pick up their feet heavily and lay them down flatly. Their knees seem to be completely cemented and stiff. There is little movement in the swinging hip motion, their spines are rigid and so are their heads. All of the elasticity and resiliency seems to have gone out of what should be a free-swinging body.

39

Crystals Are Cement Not Lubrication

Between the moveable joints of every bone in the human body, Mother Nature has placed an abundant supply of a lubricant known as synovial fluid. Take a look at a youngster who is, say 10 years of age, and watch the easy movement of every moveable joint in his body. **Why is this?** I know that your answer would be, "This child is only 10 years of age. I am 66. I can't have the same freedom of motion in my joints as a child of 10 does." My answer to you is, "Why can't you? Years have nothing to do with the amount of synovial fluid that allows the joints to move freely and easily. There is just one thing that cements your body's moveable joints and that is the build-up of toxic acid crystals."

Age is not toxic. Just because you live 50, 60 or 70 years, there should be no diminishing of the supply of synovial fluid due to your calendar years.

The word "vegetarian" is not derived from "vegetable," but from the Latin, homo vegetus, meaning among the Romans a strong, robust, thoroughly healthy man. – Paul C. Bragg

How Toxic Acid Crystals Build in Your Body

Despite the fact that I am way past 85, I pride myself on having the most flexible body, regardless of my age, and I feel ageless! I can perform difficult yoga postures with ease while standing on my head. Few people in the world can do this regardless of age. Mother Nature can't stiffen and cement one person's body as they age and yet allow me to have the flexibility of a youngster.

There are 4 great eliminative systems in our bodies that get rid of the poisons created by our daily living. By nature, we eat food, we drink liquids and we breathe air. Most humans eat too much food, eating by habit rather than by hunger. They have been brainwashed to believe that they must have scheduled meals by the clock. I know from long experience as a Physical Therapist that people with these grotesque shapes have not been able to burn up these so-called regular meals. They have been conditioned to eat breakfast whether they have hunger or not, so they load up on ham, bacon, eggs, hot cakes, doughnuts, toast, jelly, marmalade, sweet rolls, fried potatoes, waffles, pork sausage, coffee, tea, hot chocolate and dry and cooked cereals.

The body does not have enough Vital Force to masticate, digest, assimilate and eliminate these heavy breakfasts. There is always a toxic residue left . . . where does this toxic residue go? It is concentrated and crystallized as deposits in the moveable joints in the body. It's a slow process that few sense until the joints start to give them trouble. It takes years of wrong eating to create these heavy concentrations of acid crystals and toxins in the moveable joints. When these calcium-like spurs attach themselves to the joints and calcified substances replace the synovial fluid, it's then the pains and aches are felt in the moveable joints of the body.

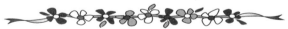

The USA leads the world in heart diseases, strokes, cancers and diabetes!

Water flows through every single part of your body, cleansing and nourishing it. But the wrong kind of water – with inorganic minerals, harmful toxins, chemicals and other contaminants can pollute, clog and gradually turn every part of your body to stone.

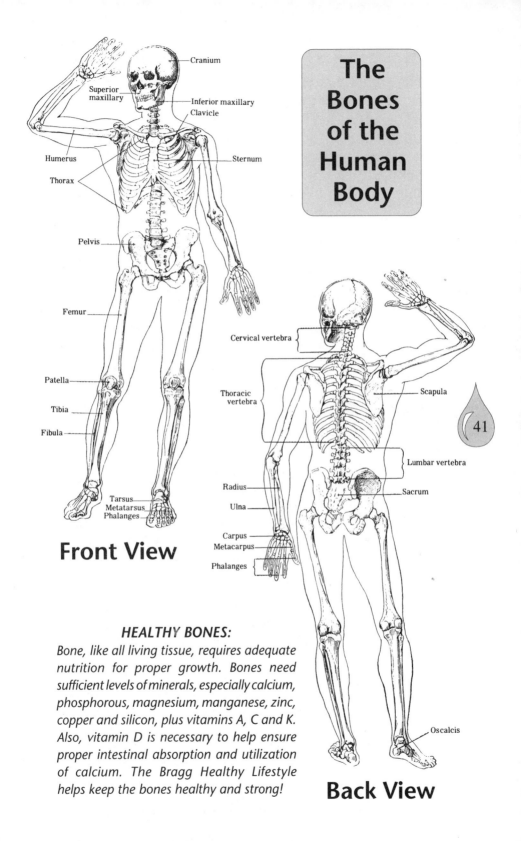

The Bones of the Human Body

Cranium

Superior maxillary

Inferior maxillary

Clavicle

Humerus

Thorax

Sternum

Pelvis

Femur

Cervical vertebra

Thoracic vertebra

Scapula

Patella

Tibia

Fibula

Lumbar vertebra

Radius

Ulna

Sacrum

Carpus

Metacarpus

Phalanges

Tarsus

Metatarsus

Phalanges

Oscalcis

41

Front View

Back View

HEALTHY BONES:

Bone, like all living tissue, requires adequate nutrition for proper growth. Bones need sufficient levels of minerals, especially calcium, phosphorous, magnesium, manganese, zinc, copper and silicon, plus vitamins A, C and K. Also, vitamin D is necessary to help ensure proper intestinal absorption and utilization of calcium. The Bragg Healthy Lifestyle helps keep the bones healthy and strong!

Back Pains – The Curse of Mankind

The toxic crystals first attack the feet, which have more than 26 moveable bones in each foot. The force of gravity sends the toxic crystals down into the feet. Gradually the feet and the ankles start to stiffen, because the toxic acid crystals are taking over and replacing the lubrication in the joints of the feet. Instead of having flexible feet, they become stiff and tire easily. They ache, burn and cause tremendous misery.

From the feet and ankles, the toxic acid crystals move upward, causing many people to suffer from pains in the knees. As time marches on, so does the deterioration of the joints. Soon toxic crystals creep into the great moveable hip joints – you will notice by the way people move their hips that they are stiff and painful.

Few people escape an aching or stiff back. Watch middle-aged people bend over and notice the agony on their faces when they straighten up. Day after day they cry out in anguish, "Oh, my aching back!" But the toxic acid crystals don't stop in the lower back, they go up into the spine, the shoulder blades, the shoulder joints, the neck and elbows . . . eventually creeping into the wrists and fingers. Some people are so full of toxic acid crystals that they cannot close their hands or make fists. They all seem to falsely blame one thing: "All my aches and pains are due to the fact that I am getting old."

Don't you believe it. These acid crystals are poisons that stayed in your body and cemented themselves in the moveable joints. Billions of pain pills are used by the American public to get relief from aching joints. Thousands of people go to hot mineral baths to get relief. Many different medical treatments are used for the relief of their problems. I am offering you The Bragg Healthy Lifestyle to help guide you onto the road to health so you can help your body heal itself.

*Make me aware that there is more
to life than measuring its speed.*

*Periodic fasting keeps you connected to your body's natural tendency
to cleanse and rejuvenate.* – Pamela Serure, *The 3-Day Energy Fast*

Fasting for Purification

When you fast for 24 to 36 hours, or from 3 to 10 days, the healing power starts to work in your body. I have told you, over and over, that the power to cleanse, purify and rejuvenate yourself is within your body. This power has always been in your body. When you go on a complete distilled water fast, the Vital Force in your body that would ordinarily be used to masticate, digest, assimilate and eliminate food is used to purify your body. That is what fasting is: deep internal cleansing, a physiological rest to build Vital Force.

Now, say you are a person of 60 and you have been eating 3 meals daily, whether you were hungry or not, and you have allowed toxic acid crystals to get deposited into the moveable joints of your body. It is going to take time for Mother Nature and the vital power within your body to break down the toxic crystals that have accumulated over the years.

The Man Who Rebuilt Himself

I remember a Mr. Evans who came to me years ago. He hobbled painfully into my office. A well known doctor in California had given him a prescription which read "Physical therapy as prescribed." I am also a physical therapist which helped in my health and healing practice.

This man's sad story is one of millions in our country. He had never been educated to know how to care for his wonderful body, but he had been conditioned to eat 3 meals per day and eat anything that pleased him. Now, I have told you several times in this book that "Human Flesh is Dumb." You can put anything in your stomach at any hour that you wish. You can get up in the morning and fill up on cereal, ham and eggs, fried potatoes and toast and wash it down with 5 cups of coffee, but you must take the consequences of eating habits like this.

There is only one water that is clean and that is steam distilled water. No other substance on our planet does so much to keep us healthy and get us well as this distilled water does. – Dr. James F. Balch, MD, Dietary Wellness

Victory Won By Fasting, Diet and Exercise

First and foremost, your body has to earn its food by the sweat of your brow. That means you only eat food appropriate to your physical activity and climate. This man was eating as he did when he was a young active farm boy. Slowly his joints were becoming cemented solid by toxins and toxic crystals that were pressing on nerves causing him agonizing pain. He wanted an easy way out of his misery. I told him truthfully that it had taken a long time of wrong eating and bad habits of living to get him in this wretched condition. Now it would take fasting, a healthy diet and ample exercises to help relieve these pains. He was an intelligent man and saw the truth of my simple philosophy.

I started him on a 3 day distilled water fast. Following the fast, I had him eat only fresh fruit for breakfast and a raw vegetable combination salad for lunch. I had him eat a grated carrot, beet, chopped cabbage salad and one cooked vegetable for dinner. I took him off all animal products, meat, fish, eggs, cheese and dairy products. I eliminated all salt, sugar and refined foods. I took him off all grains and all legumes such as beans, peas, rice and lentils for two months. Every day I had him take a 10 minute hot bath (add 1 cup apple cider vinegar), bringing the water up to 104 degrees, using a bath thermometer. I gave him an exercise program of brisk walking starting with 3 blocks the first day, and every third day I added another block to his walking program until he was walking 3 miles a day.

Every week he took a 36 hour water fast. As the days and weeks rolled into months, I gave him one 7 day and one 10 day fast. In one year you would hardly have recognized this man! His family and friends were amazed at his transformation. His joints became flexible and, although he hadn't been swimming for years, he joined the YMCA and swam 3 days a week. He hadn't ridden a bicycle for years, yet he purchased one and rode for miles at a time. He and his wife took up dancing and in a year he was winning contests. The stiffness left him. He even took up the piano and became a good piano player.

Mother Nature Works Miracles Slowly, But Surely When You Honor Her Laws

Mr. Evans is growing younger as he is growing older. His miseries are gone! He accomplished all this by himself! I only helped him to help himself! As a health teacher, I only laid out his healthy lifestyle program of natural living. Today he fasts every week for 24 to 36 hours without fail. Four times a year – winter, spring, summer and fall – he takes a 10 day complete fast. His lively steps are that of a man 20 years of age! His movements are quick and accurate. He didn't do all this in a day, in a week or a month. It took time to break down and eliminate the poisons and toxic acid crystals that were tormenting him.

What Mr. Evans did you can do too! The body is self-repairing, self-healing and self-maintaining. All you have to do is live by the laws of God and Mother Nature, and you will be rewarded with the joy of living.

Be a faithful health captain and live The Bragg Healthy Lifestyle! I don't want you to have to totter along on life-support drug cocktails and hip replacements, but choose to LIVE with super energy and total health!

Fasting is an important part of your program for banishing toxic acid crystals from the moveable joints of your body. You and only you know how free your joints are of this toxic material which causes premature ageing. Start today on your first 24 hour, distilled water fast. You be the judge of what effects fasting will have on the many moveable joints of your body. At this very second, roll your head round and round. Do you hear that grating, grinding sound toxic acid crystals?

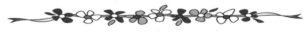

To lengthen thy life, lessen thy meals. – Ben Franklin

Enter – or perhaps re-enter – the brave new world of wellness through exercise, natural remedies, alternative therapies, meditation and positive thinking.
– Monica Skrzypczak

The body must be nourished, physically, emotionally and spiritually. We're spiritually starved in America and not underfed but undernourished.
– Carol Hornig

Toxic Acid Crystals Make Joints Grind

The grinding sound you hear is the toxic acid crystals that have deposited themselves on the uppermost bone of your spine – the Atlas. Your 24 hour or 7 day fast will not eliminate all the toxic acid crystals from your Atlas, but the body purification will be started. Fast one day a week. In one year you will have fasted 52 days. In that time the Vital Force of your body will have dissolved a large amount of the acid crystals from your joints.

Each time you fast you will notice more freedom in every joint in your body. A feeling of agelessness will replace that tight, stiff, ageing feeling. Once again you will feel free and loose in every moveable joint of your body. You will have Mother Nature, fasting and eating natural food to thank for your "New Youthful Feeling!"

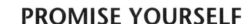

PROMISE YOURSELF

- *To be so strong that nothing can disturb your peace of mind.*
- *To talk health, happiness, prosperity to every person you meet.*
- *To make all your friends feel that they are special.*
- *To look at the sunny side of everything and make your optimism come true.*
- *To think only of the best, work only for the best and expect only the best.*
- *To be just as enthusiastic about the success of others as you are about yours.*
- *To forget the mistakes of the past and press on to the greater achievements of the bright, fresh future.*
- *To wear a cheerful countenance at all times and give every living creature you meet a smile.*
- *To give so much time to the improvements of yourself that you have no time to be critical of others.*
- *To be too large for worry, too strong for fear, too noble for anger, and too happy to permit the presence of trouble.*

– Christian D. Larson

Chapter 5

Scientific Fasting Explained

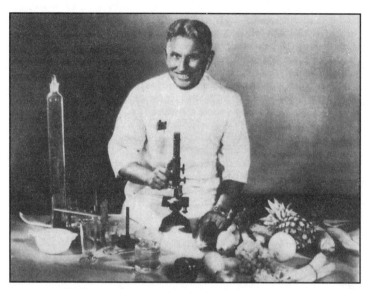

Paul C. Bragg – Fasting & Life Extension Specialist

Fasting has been practiced by man and animals since the beginning of time. Primitive man had no other method of healing except fasting. He would fast when he got hurt or when ill, because fasting was a natural instinct for self preservation. Along with fasting, he used herbs from the field and forest as tonics and antiseptics.

I believe that fasting is Mother Nature's best remedy! For, as we will see, properly conducted fasts purify the body, restoring it to health after everything has failed.

In over 70 years of supervising fasts, I have seen miracles happen to people who were ready for the human scrap yard that truly could be called miraculous. Fasting is not only the oldest method of fighting physical problems, but the best of all remedies because it has no side effects. Fasting is the most natural and original process of cleansing and purifying the body.

Fasting is the greatest remedy – the physician within!
– Paracelsus, 15th century physician.
He established the role of chemistry in medicine.

Fasting is as Old as Man

The instinct that leads us to fast when the body is sick or wounded resides in the cells of every living being. The reason sick or wounded animals refuse to eat is that the instinct of self-preservation takes away their hunger so they will not eat. In this way, the Vital Force (which would otherwise have to be used in the digestion of food) is concentrated at the site of the injury to remove waste products, thus purifying and healing the body. The fasting instinct is so powerful and of such vital importance that, even though semi-civilized man has strayed from the natural path, he is still greatly influenced by this wonderful saving scheme of Mother Nature! If he would obey the silent voice of this infallible, natural instinct and stop eating when hunger has been withdrawn, he would soon get well. Better still, he would never get sick again, provided he ate natural food, lived in a natural environment and lived a sane, sensible, healthy and natural life.

Since the infallible intelligence of the living organism withdraws the sensation of hunger when there is an excess of food or when the body has been wounded, the desire to fast begins when either of these happen.

We read in ancient history that fasting has been practiced since time immemorial by the religious people of the East and by most ancient civilizations. They practiced fasting not only for the recovery of health and preservation of youth, but for spiritual illumination as well. Accordingly, we see the great philosopher, Pythagoras, requiring his disciples to undertake a fast of 40 days before they could be initiated into the mysteries of his philosophical teachings. He claimed that only through a 40 day fast could the minds of his disciples by sufficiently purified and clarified to understand the profound teachings of the mysteries of life.

As it was in the old days, fasting will not only purify the body and help restore it to well-being, but has a great effect on the mental and spiritual parts of man.

Mother Nature and its beauty is the signature of God.

Fasting Awakens the Mind and Soul

In my own personal life, as well as in the lives of many of my students who have been conscientious and persistent in their fasting program, great mental and spiritual doors have been opened! If I read a book today, my mind retains what I read as clearly as if the book were in front of me . . . that is, I have a photographic memory. Hundreds of my students write that they, too, have developed a keen photographic mind. After a fast of 1 to 3 days, you will notice that a dark cloud has been lifted out of your mind. You can think more logically and you can come to decisions quite quickly. What was once a great problem becomes trivial! After a fast, you seem to fear nothing any more and things you worried about are solved easily by your purified mind.

In my personal life, fasting helped me develop a keen extrasensory perception. I can find solutions for many problems that once caused me many hours of anxiety and nerve-exhausting worrying. My fasting program has created an inner peaceful tranquillity of mind. I feel more serene and at peace with myself and the world because of my continued fasting program. As you purify your body and mind, you seem to come closer to a power higher than yourself! This inner strength and inner power, makes you a positive-thinking person.

The memory becomes sharp as a razor's edge. You can remember names, places and events that go back many years. You have a better capacity for self-education. Education is not a preparation for life, but education is life itself! To grow mentally and spiritually is the greatest goal we humans can have on this earth. So fasting works three ways. You purify your body physically, mentally and spiritually and therefore enjoy super vitality and health. Your mind becomes a sponge which can absorb new facts and knowledge. Greatest of all are the inner peacefulness and spiritual tranquillity that make life worth living. Through fasting you find "Peace of Mind," the greatest and rarest gift of life.

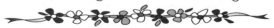

You are encircled by the arms of the mystery of God. – Hildegard of Bingen

The Biblical Patriarchs Fasted

We know that in ancient times, the patriarchs of the Bible fasted frequently. Moses, Elijah, David and others fasted for as long as 40 days. We know that Christ fasted 40 days before he began to teach the great truths of life. We read in the Bible that Christ sent forth his disciples after saying to them, "Heal the sick, cleanse the leper, raise the dead, cast out devils, freely ye have received, freely give." At the same time, Christ knew that there were dangers awaiting those who dared to bring truth to the people. Therefore, Christ warned his disciples with these words, "Behold! I send you forth as sheep in the midst of wolves: be ye therefore wise as serpents and harmless as doves." (Matthew 10: 8,16)

As in the olden days, there are dispensers of gloom, fear, and destruction when the subject of fasting is brought up today. I have heard people discuss how unscientific fasting is and when I asked them if they had ever fasted, they gave me a definite answer "Never!"

These dispensers of gloom still cling to the old idea that you must eat to keep up your strength, and that when you stop eating, you collapse. This is far from the truth! A little discomfort which may occur during fasting only happens because we are creatures of habit. If we are able to handle the first 3 days of fasting, then it becomes easier. You lose your appetite and craving for food. Your energy level increases and your mind gets sharper and moves faster!

Accuse not nature, she hath done her part; do thou but thine. – Milton, *Paradise Lost*

Fasting is a normal part of our walk with God, as is exemplified by the Lord Jesus. Immediately following the Lord's Prayer, He said: Moreover when ye fast, be not of sad countenance, that thou appear not unto men to fast, but unto thy Father, which is in secret and thy Father shall reward thee openly. – Matthew 6:16 -18

To preserve health is a moral and religious duty, for health is the basis for all social virtues. We can no longer be as useful when not well. – Dr. Samuel Johnson, Father of Dictionaries

Fasting – The Safe, Perfect Cleanser

Of course, if you are loaded with toxic poisons, fasting will flush these poisons out of the body and you will feel a little uncomfortable, but these are momentary experiences and should cause no concern. This means only that fasting is working for you. You know you are fasting to purify the body of the accumulated toxic poisons and waste. When you feel uncomfortable, you can say to yourself, "This is only temporary. This will pass as soon as these old toxins are flushed out of my body." And what miracle rewards you'll receive for the small, temporary discomfort you may have experienced.

Your eyes become brighter and all the natural senses of the body seem to be sharper! After a fast, your food tastes better – the fruits and the vegetables taste so marvelous, because of your newly revitalized taste sense! Your body seems to be tireless and you will sleep like a baby after a fast. There are so many rewards from a fast that only a person who has actually fasted can truly realize the great benefits that are achieved.

Don't be a Slave to Foods

Most humans are slaves to foods; they must have breakfast, lunch and dinner at regular meal hours every day, year in and year out. They eat whether they are hungry or not, and their poor bodies are burdened by overeating . . . and usually poor nutrition as well! No wonder we have so many physical wrecks! One of the greatest nutritional teachers in the world, Professor Arnold Ehret, said, "Life is a tragedy of nutrition." How true is the old trite saying, "Man digs his grave with his knife and fork!" Many people never give their stomachs a rest. They continually stuff and work the digestive and eliminative functions with an overabundance of food. This excessive burden means that the functions of digestion and elimination become so overworked and so exhausted that they simply collapse. The entire body then becomes enervated! Millions suffer from fatigue.

Old age is not a time of life. It is a condition of the body. It is not time that ages the body, it is abuse that does. – Herbert Shelton

Fasting Program Regularly Removes Toxins

After a fast, you will find you don't need as much food as you used to eat! The fast shrinks your stomach and you will feel lighter, look better and have more vitality on ½ the food you were accustomed to.

I am an active man physically, yet I eat only two light meals daily. I never snack between meals. Nibbling and compulsory eating have been eliminated from my life by my years of the 24 hour weekly fast and my fasts lasting from 7 to 10 days, 3 or 4 times a year. After the fast, your eyes sparkle and your skin tone improves. Notice the more energy and vitality you have. Your heart sings a lighthearted song because your body is cleaner and healthier. It's not burdened with fighting toxic poisons. Your fasting program keeps lifting the toxins from your bloodstream and vital organs regularly.

Plan Your Fasting Program Today

So if you want to enjoy all these great benefits, be a strong positive person, plan a fasting program for yourself, and live strictly by it. Don't tell anyone you are going to fast, because the average person is ignorant of the facts of fasting and they are not qualified to criticize your health program. I never discuss my fasting with people who have no knowledge of the miracles of fasting. Why should I discuss it with them? They are still full of fears held by the average person; that if they miss a few meals, they will starve to death. So be intelligent enough not to tell others what you are doing. You will simply get a lot of worthless advice. Many times while I am fasting for a week I conduct large Health Crusades and I tell no one I am on a complete fast. Your fasting time is very personal and it belongs to you, not to anyone else. If you have faith in it, that's all that's necessary. You are putting faith in God and Mother Nature's oldest and most respected way of purifying, renovating and rejuvenating your body – fasting!

Many dishes, many diseases. – Ben Franklin

If mankind profits from its mistakes, we have a glorious future ahead of us!

Your Mind Must Rule Your Body
To Fast Successfully

Remember, "Flesh is dumb!" It has no intelligence or reasoning power. If, after reading this book, you are convinced, without any reservations, that a fasting program is going to elevate you to greater heights of living, then your mind becomes the master of your flesh. Your mind must be stronger than the desires of your flesh, because your body has long been conditioned to have food put into it at various intervals of the day.

The average person gets up and eats breakfast whether hungry or not. When the stomach does all the directing, the mind tags along with it's desires. So, through reflex conditioning, the stomach expects food for breakfast. To me, breakfast is a worthless meal. The body has been at rest all night. It has not expended energy, so why should a person get up after the inactivity of sleep and put a big breakfast into the stomach? I will tell you again, "You must earn your food with physical activity!"

53

No Breakfast Plan is Best

Another reason why I am a believer and a follower of the No Breakfast Plan is because big breakfasts drain and exhaust most people of the energy that has been gathered by the night's sleep. In the morning, your energy – physical, mental, and spiritual – should be at its highest. With this new energy that the body has created, you can do great creative and physical work.

I have shown elementary school students and high school students and college students that they can do their greatest studying early in the morning on an empty stomach. Most students eat an evening meal, which is their heaviest meal of the day, and then they try to study.

It's a terrific effort to concentrate and study after eating a huge dinner! Why does this happen? It seems that the mind just will not work after a heavy meal. But give these same students a good night's rest, get them up early in the morning and keep food out of them for 2 or 3 hours and they will become brilliant students.

I have taught this no breakfast plan to millions of our health followers and readers around the world. This is the logical reason why I don't believe in a heavy breakfast. A heavy meal requires most of the total nerve energy of the body to handle digestion, thus the mind becomes enervated, making people dull, sleepy and leaving the precious nerve energy at its lowest ebb.

Let's look at it from another standpoint. Through long years of misinformation, people have been told, "Breakfast is the most important meal of the day. It gives you the strength, the energy and the vitality to do a hard morning's work, either physically or mentally." This is absolutely erroneous! It is not a true scientific fact. When you eat a heavy breakfast, through reflex action you feel full and satisfied, but you do not gain strength. It takes hours for this food to be processed by the digestive system before you can gain any energy or vitality from a big breakfast. Digestion is a most complicated process. Every item of food in the breakfast has to be broken down into fine chemical fragments so that the cells of the body are fed.

You Must Earn Your Food by Exercising

You can plainly see that healthy eating is a matter of conditioning and habit. I haven't eaten breakfast for over 65 years. I get up early every morning. When at our Hollywood home, I drive to the beautiful Griffith Park mountain trail and hike for several hours up to the top of Mt. Hollywood and top it off by running down the mountain. If I am at our home near Malibu, Patricia and I take long hikes and runs on the beach. I am not only a summer swimmer, but a year-round ocean swimmer. At our desert home, we hike the hills and ride our bicycles. After several hours of vigorous exercise, we return home to enjoy our fruit meal. Now we are ready to do our best creative work, planning the Bragg Health Crusades, writing articles for health magazines or writing our health books to inspire you to become healthier!

Eat to live, not live to eat. – Ben Franklin

Healthy Eating Habits Keep You Youthful

Around noon or so we will eat our main meal of the day. We start with a large delicious salad, (recipe pg. 231). After the salad we have one cooked yellow vegetable – such as a baked yam or carrots – one green vegetable, such as Swiss chard, kale, mustard greens, broccoli, zucchini, squash or green beans – and some type of vegetable protein. We enjoy tofu, beans, lentils and raw unsalted nuts of all kinds and seeds, such as sunflower, pumpkin, sesame, etc. (Vegetable Protein Chart pg. 233).

Patricia and I have earned this meal through exercise. Now our bodies are ready to send forth the digestive juices and the internal secretions to get all of the nourishment and energy out of this natural food. The digestive juices of the mouth and stomach are abundant. As an extra benefit, regular exercise, ample fresh fruits and healthy salads promote good elimination.

This program of 12 meals a week, 2 meals per day, 6 days a week does not burden and exhaust the body's digestive system and the bowel eliminative powers of the body (we fast for one 24 to 36 hour period weekly). On this Bragg Healthy Lifestyle program, you don't overeat, you educate your bowels to move soon upon arising. Usually you will have a bowel evacuation within an hour after lunch and an hour after the evening meal.

The only exception we ever make for snacking between meals is to have some luscious, juicy organic fruit. In mid-afternoon, we have a juicy organic apple or fresh pineapple, mango or papaya. When melons are in season, we find nothing more refreshing than sweet, ripe melons; particularly watermelon, cantaloupe, honeydew or casaba.

Most people are sick or half sick most of the time. It is our opinion that they enervate their body and exhaust themselves in trying to burn up all those extra calories from all the excess foods they consume!

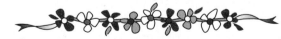

You can't put a monetary value on life, it's priceless!
Our health is the motivator of our lives! Guard and
treasure life by living The Bragg Healthy Lifestyle!

Americans Love to Eat Socially!

The main reason why 65% to 70% of Americans are overweight is because eating has become a fun, social gorging event! People eat breakfast, eat at the coffee break, eat at lunch and eat at their afternoon coffee break. They eat a large dinner and long before the big dinner can be handled by the digestive system they are eating again, plus drinking alcohol, colas or coffee while watching TV. No wonder they are constantly tired! It's because they enervate themselves by exhausting their Vital Force. Even the healthiest person only generates so much Vital Force daily and, if by over-eating habits or other bad habits you exhaust your Vital Force, then there is not sufficient energy for the needed work of mastication, digestion, metabolism and elimination.

What happens? There is not enough Vital Force to flush the waste out of the body, so this stockpiles and concentrates and that's how you build autointoxication. Your troubles and premature ageing start right here!

Keeping Internally Clean is Critical

Sickness and premature ageing are no mystery. You are punished by your bad habits, not for them! If you keep stuffing food that cannot be handled into your over loaded digestive tract, it only rots, putrefies and poisons the billions of your body's cells. You are sick, weak and prematurely old because you have not learned how to keep your body clean inside! The secret of health and long life can be summed up in three words: "Keep Clean Inside!" Etch these words of wisdom deep on the blackboard of your brain! Repeat them over and over again as an affirmation . . . "Keep Clean Inside!"

Fasting is the best and most natural way of cleansing, purifying and rejuvenating your body because it is Mother Nature's natural method. Nobody can do it for you. It is a personal matter. It costs you nothing but a strong, positive willpower! Remember, woe to the weak. Life is the survival of the fittest . . . and fasting is a program of self-preservation!

Remember always, you are punished by your bad habits of living, not for them, but by them! – Paul C. Bragg

Are You Ready to Fast, Detox and Get Healthy?

If you are convinced, without reservation that fasting is a time to get detoxed and healthy, then you're ready. Remember, when you tell your conscious and your subconscious mind you're going to fast for internal purity you set things in motion for success! You have told every cell in your body that a fast is going to improve your health. Your body's cells will accept this command.

Start with a 24 hour distilled water fast. During these 24 hours you are going to put nothing into your stomach except distilled water. If you eat fruit with this, it is not a fast; it is a fruit diet. If you drink fruit or vegetable juices during this 24 hour period it ceases to be a complete fast, and instead becomes either a vegetable or fruit juice fast. I want you to bear this in mind: a complete fast is nothing allowed in the stomach except distilled water! Your first fast may be easy or it may have some rough spots. You may fast from lunch to lunch or dinner to dinner, as long as you abstain from food for an entire 24 hours. If you are accustomed to coffee, tea, beer or alcohol drinks, you might have reactions . . . one typical reaction appears in the form of a headache.

Why does this happen? Because the cells of your body have conditioned themselves to regular dosages of a stimulant. When you take the stimulant away from the nerves and the cells there is bound to be a reaction. But remember, this fast is going to help break that stimulant habit, because during the 24 hour distilled water fast you are flushing many of the buried poisonous residues out of your body through your eliminative organs.

During their 24 hour fast, most people can carry on their regular duties, even though they may have a little discomfort. There may be some turbulence in the stomach but, all in all, it should go smoothly and successfully if you make your mind be master of your flesh. You are giving the commands to your body from your higher brain cells. You're not going to be dragged down to the level of the lower stomach cells. Remember it's important everyday, especially fast days, to drink ample water. Get started!

Juice Fast – an Introduction to Water Fast

Fasting has been rediscovered through juice fasting — as a simple, easy means of cleansing and restoring health and vitality. To fast (abstain from food) comes from the Old English word *fasten* or *to hold firm*. It's a means to commit oneself to the task of finding inner strength through body, mind and soul cleansing. Throughout history the world's greatest philosophers and sages, including Socrates, Plato, Buddha and Gandhi, have enjoyed fasting and preached its benefits.

Juice bars are springing up everywhere and juice fasting has become "in" with the theatrical crowd in Hollywood, New York and in London. The number of Stars who believe in the power and effectiveness of juice and water fasting is growing. A partial list includes Steven Spielberg, George Hamilton, Barbra Streisand, Kim Basinger, Alec Baldwin, Daryl Hannah, Christie Brinkley, Madonna, Goldie Hawn, Donna Karan and many other Hollywood Stars. They say fasting helps balance their lives physically, mentally and emotionally.

Although a pure water fast is best, an introductory liquid juice fast can offer people an ideal opportunity to give their intestinal systems a restful, cleansing relief from the commercial high-fat, high-sugar, high-salt and high-protein fast foods most Americans exist on.

Organic, raw, live fruit and vegetable juices can be purchased fresh from many Health Food Stores. You can also prepare these healthy juices yourself using a good home juicer. When juice fasting, it's best to dilute the juice with ⅓ distilled water. This juice combination list gives you many varieties. With vegetable and tomato combinations try adding a dash of Bragg Liquid Aminos, herbs or, on non-fast days, even some green powder (barley, chlorella, spirulina, etc.) to create a delicious, nutritious powerful health drink. When using herbs in these drinks, use 1 to 2 fresh leaves or a tiny pinch of dried herbs. A pinch of dulse (seaweed) rich in protein, iodine and iron – is delicious with vegetable juices.

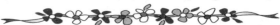

To work the head, temperance must be carried into the diet. – Beecher

Here are Some Powerful Juice Combinations:

1. Beet, celery, alfalfa sprouts
2. Cabbage, celery and apple
3. Cabbage, cucumber, celery, tomato, spinach and basil
4. Tomato, carrot and mint
5. Carrot, celery, watercress, garlic and wheatgrass
6. Grapefruit, orange and lemon
7. Beet, parsley, celery, carrot, cabbage and garlic
8. Beet, celery, dulse and carrot
9. Cucumber, carrot and parsley
10. Watercress, cucumber, garlic
11. Asparagus, carrot, and mint
12. Carrot, celery, parsley, onion, cabbage and sweet basil
13. Carrot and coconut milk
14. Carrot, broccoli, lemon, cayenne
15. Carrot, cauliflower, rosemary
16. Apple, carrot, radish, ginger
17. Apple, pineapple and mint
18. Apple, papaya and grapes
19. Papaya, cranberries and apple
20. Leafy greens, broccoli, apple
21. Grape, cherry and apple
22. Watermelon (include seeds)

Juicing has come a long way since Paul C. Bragg imported the first hand operated vegetable-fruit juicer from Germany and introduced juice therapy to America. Before this, juice was pressed by hand using cheesecloth. Juices are now considered an ideal health beverage worldwide!

Fruit bears the closest relation to light. The sun pours a continuous flood of light into the fruits, and they furnish the best potion of food a human being requires for the sustenance of mind and body. –Alcott

59

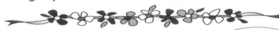

Bad Nutrition – #1 Cause of Sickness

"Diet-related diseases account for 68% of all deaths."

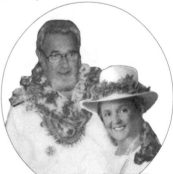

Dr. Koop & Patricia

Dr. C. Everett Koop, our friend and America's former Surgeon General said this in his famous 1988 landmark report on nutrition and health in America. People don't die of infectious conditions as such, but of malnutrition that allows the germs to get a foothold in sickly bodies. Also, bad nutrition is usually the main cause of noninfectious, fatal or degenerative conditions. When the body has its full vitamin and mineral quota, including precious potassium, it's almost impossible for germs to get a foothold in a healthy, powerful bloodstream and tissues!

The 70% Watery Human

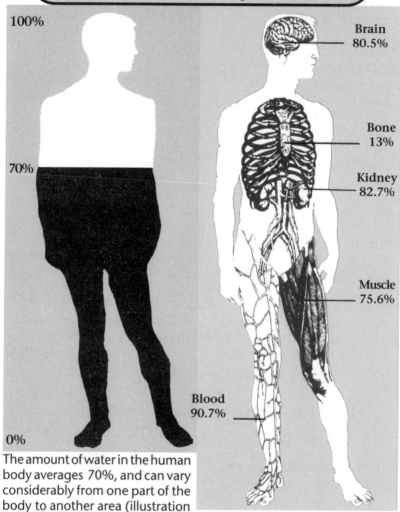

100%

Brain
80.5%

Bone
13%

70%

Kidney
82.7%

Muscle
75.6%

Blood
90.7%

60

0%

The amount of water in the human body averages 70%, and can vary considerably from one part of the body to another area (illustration on right). A lean man may hold 70% of his weight in body water, while a woman – because of her larger proportion of water-poor fatty tissues – may be only 52% water. The lowering of the water content in the blood is what triggers the hypothalamus, the brain's thirst center, to send out its familiar urgent demand for a drink of water.

Water Percentage in Various Body Parts:

Teeth	10%	Lungs	80%
Bones	13%	Brain	80.5%
Cartilage	55%	Bile	86%
Red blood corpuscles	68.7%	Plasma	90%
Liver	71.5%	Blood	90.7%
Muscle tissue	75%	Lymph	94%
Spleen	75.5%	Saliva	95.5%

Chapter 6

Why I Drink Only Distilled Water!

When I refer to fasting in this book, I constantly make the statement, "Eat absolutely no food and drink distilled water exclusively." Distilled water is pure H_2O – which means it's a compound of 2 parts hydrogen and 1 part oxygen. If you drink rain water, or the fresh juices of fruits and vegetables, remember that all of this liquid has been distilled by Mother Nature. If you drink rain water or snow water, there are no inorganic minerals in it. It is 100% mineral-free. If you drink fruit and vegetable juices, you are drinking distilled water plus certain nutrients such as fruit sugars, organic minerals and vitamins. But if you drink lake, river, well or spring water, you are drinking undistilled water, plus the inorganic minerals that the water has picked up. Some of this water is known as hard water, meaning it has high inorganic mineral concentrations that can cause health problems.

61

Now, let me give you a short lesson in chemistry. There are two kinds of chemicals - inorganic and organic. The inorganic chemicals are inert, which means that they cannot be absorbed into the tissues of the body.

Our bodies are composed of 16 organic minerals which all come from that which is living or was alive. When we eat an apple or any other fruit or vegetable, that substance is living. Each has a certain survival time after it has been picked before spoiling. We prefer the vegetarian diet, but the same applies to animal foods, fish, milk, cheese and eggs if you eat them.

Dehydration of certain organs will result in symptoms which are often misdiagnosed by physicians. The message is: drink your way to health with volumes of pure water. – F. Batmanghelidj, M.D. author of *Your Body's Many Cries for Water; You Are Not Sick, You Are Thirsty!*

Hard, Inorganic Minerals Cause Problems!

Organic minerals are very vital in keeping us alive and well. If we were cast away on an uninhabited island where nothing was growing, we would starve to death. Even though the soil beneath our feet contains 16 inorganic minerals, our bodies could not absorb them. Only a living plant has the power to extract inorganic minerals from the earth. No human can extract the nourishment from inorganic minerals.

Many years ago, I was on an expedition to China when one part of the country was suffering from drought and famine. I saw with my own eyes poor, starving people heating earth and eating it for want of food. They died horrible deaths because they could not get one bit of nourishment from the inorganic minerals of the earth.

For years I have heard people say that certain waters were rich in all the minerals. What minerals are they talking about? Inorganic or organic? These are inorganic and they are burdening their bodies with these inert minerals, which may cause the development of stones in the kidneys, gallbladder and stone-like acid crystals in the arteries, veins, and other parts of the body.

I was reared in Virginia where the drinking water is called hard water. It is heavily saturated with inorganic minerals, especially sodium, iron and calcium. I saw many of my elders die of kidney troubles. Nearly all the people were prematurely old because the inorganic minerals would collect on the inner walls of their arteries and veins, causing many to die from hardening of the arteries, strokes and heart attacks. One of my uncles died at Johns Hopkins hospital when he was only 48. The autopsy doctors stated that his arteries were as hard as clay pipes because they were so stiff and corroded with inorganic minerals.

Yet you will hear people say, "Distilled water is dead water. A fish cannot live in it." Of course a fish cannot live in freshly distilled water for any length of time, because it needs the vegetation that grows in rivers, lakes and seas. Imagine you were shipwrecked while on a passenger ship going to Hawaii and you became a castaway in a lifeboat for days on the open sea. If the only water available was rain water, would you say, "Rain water is dead distilled water, I won't drink it?" No, you would never say that. Of course you would drink it and survive until rescued!

Millions Drink Rain (Distilled) Water!

By drinking distilled water, you would be joining millions worldwide who drink unpolluted rain water. Man evolved drinking rain water. In Bermuda, etc., where soil is so porous that water cannot be held in the soil, people have special roofs to catch rain water so that it drains into tanks under their houses or nearby.

The great castle of the powerful emperor Tiberius, who ruled the world at the time of Christ, is located on the Isle of Capri. It has a remarkable reservoir to catch rain water inside the castle walls. Today, 2000 years later, the people of Capri still go to this reservoir for water during a dry spell. I have seen this with my own eyes, you can too!

Years ago, when the great actor Douglas Fairbanks, Sr., and I were close friends, we roamed the South Sea Islands. During that trip, we came upon an island inhabited by beautiful, healthy Polynesians who never drank anything but distilled water, because the island was surrounded by the Pacific Ocean. Sea water is undrinkable because of its high salt content. Their island was based on porous coral which could not hold water, so they only had Mother Nature's distilled water drinks from rain water and fresh coconut milk.

I have never seen any finer specimens of men or women than these native South Sea Islanders! There were several doctors on the yacht who thoroughly examined the oldest people on these islands, and the heart doctor stated that he had never examined such well-preserved people in his life. They never celebrated birthdays, so they were gloriously ageless, not only in years, but in body! These older men performed as well in the vigorous native dances as the younger men. These people were beautiful specimens of humanity, and they all lived their lengthy lives drinking only Mother Nature's distilled water.

Distilled Water is Best for Your Health

Years ago, during an expedition to the Atlas mountains of Morocco, I found vigorous people roaming the desert, and the only water they drank was unpolluted rain water.

Every liquid prescription that is compounded in any drug store the world over is prepared with distilled water. It is not true that distilled water leaches the organic minerals out of the body nor is it dead water. It is the purest and safest water that man can drink!

Distilled water helps to dissolve the terrible, toxic poisons that collect in people's bodies. It passes through the kidneys without leaving inorganic pebbles and stones. If you wash your hair in rain (distilled) water you will discover the softness of soft water.

No new water has been created on the face of the earth since it was originally formed. Just as the same energy is formed and reformed, so the same water is re-used over and over again by the miracle of Mother Nature. Waters of the earth are purified by natural distillation. The sun evaporates the water. It is collected into clouds and the clouds become full and then we have rain and dew . . . pure, perfectly clean water, one of God's and Mother Nature's great miracles! Who dares to say that they supply man with dead water! Distilled water is the purest water on earth and it's free of all harmful inorganic minerals and toxic substances.

Over 70 years ago, I predicted that some day man would need clean, pure water so desperately that great government distillation plants would have to be installed at the seas to convert the unlimited supply of salt water into pure water for all purposes. I have lived to see my prediction come true. Even Santa Barbara had to build a plant during a long dry spell. In the American Navy, there are huge aircraft carriers with five thousand Navy personnel aboard. These ships cannot carry enough land water so they distill sea water for the men to drink and bathe in. Also big ocean cruise ships distill sea water for their passengers' use, bathing, etc.

Bragg Family Uses Only Distilled Water

At our Bragg homes, distilled water is delivered in 5 gallon bottles for household use. I also have it at the Bragg Santa Barbara office. Distilled water can be bought almost everywhere. It is used for baby formulas, heart and kidney patients and many other purposes.

Millions of homes across the nation have water softeners for household uses, because hard water is not good for washing clothes and it spots dishes. But please don't drink water from water softeners! It's not a healthful drinking water. Drink only distilled water exclusively for a year and you'll never drink hard or softened water again. When you fast, please use only distilled water for greater cleansing and health. Read the Bragg book – *Water – The Shocking Truth* for more info.

65

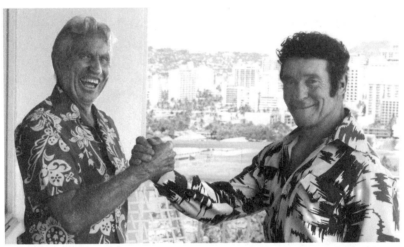

Paul C. Bragg clasps hands with Jack LaLanne

Jack says, "Bragg saved my life at age 15 when I attended the Bragg Health and Fitness Crusade in Oakland, California." From that day on Jack has lived The Bragg Healthy Lifestyle and has inspired millions to Health and Fitness.

To resist old age creeping in one must work with the body, mind, soul and the heart. And to keep strong and healthy one must live a healthy lifestyle.

It's magnificent to live long if one keeps healthy and youthful. – Harry Fosdick

Ten Common Sense Reasons Why You Should Only Drink Pure, Distilled Water!

- There are over 12,000 toxic chemicals on the market today . . . and 500 are being added yearly! Regardless of where you live, in the city or on the farm, some of these chemicals are getting into your drinking water.

- No one on the face of the earth today knows what effect these chemicals could have upon the body as they blend into thousands of different combinations. It is like making a mixture of colors; one drop could change the color.

- The equipment hasn't been designed to detect some of these chemicals and may not be for many years to come.

- The body is made up of approximately 70% water. Therefore, don't you think you should be particular about the type of water you drink?

- The Navy has been drinking distilled water for years!

- Distilled water is chemical and mineral free. Distillation removes all the chemicals and impurities from water that are possible to remove. If distillation doesn't remove them, there is no known method today that will.

- The body does need minerals . . . but it is not necessary that they come from water. There is not one mineral in water which cannot be found more abundantly in food! Water is the most unreliable source of minerals because it varies from one area to another. The food we eat – not the water we drink – is the best source of organic minerals!

- Distilled water is used for intravenous feeding, inhalation therapy, prescriptions and baby formulas. Therefore, doesn't it make common sense that it is good for everyone?

- Thousands of water distillers have been sold throughout the United States and around the world to individuals, families, dentists, doctors, hospitals, nursing homes and government agencies . . . and these informed, alert consumers are helping protect their health by using only pure, steam distilled water.

- With all of the chemicals, pollutants and other impurities in our water, it only makes good common sense you should clean up the water you drink Mother Nature's inexpensive way through distillation.

Chapter 7

How Long Should One Fast?

For a person who has no fasting experience, the longest fast should never be over 10 days, unless they are under the supervision of a health expert with fasting experience. Fasting is the most natural method of purifying the body and is truly a miracle! In my opinion, it's best to do shorter fasts for the first few months, gradually working into longer fasts. This helps prevent distress to your body by gently loosening and passing the stored toxins out of the body.

A long fast must be supervised by an expert because only they can best determine when a fast should be broken. Sometimes even the experts cannot tell how long a fast should last. When and how to break the fast is determined by carefully watching how conditions in the faster's body change during the fast. The expert watches to see how fast the body, kidneys, etc. are throwing off mucus and toxins. They will examine the urine daily – if too many toxins are being eliminated, causing a strain on the kidneys, they will usually stop the fast.

Even the greatest experts won't all agree with putting a person on a 30 or 40 day fast. Often people plan a longer fast and find toxins pouring out so quickly that it's best they do short fasts and not one big long fast. Sometimes in the first 6 days, if too many toxic poisons were released into their circulation, I felt it wise to have them stop the fast and do another short fast in a few weeks.

I have heard unqualified people say, "the long fast is best." This I do not believe, because man is the sickest creature on earth! None of God's other creatures have violated His nutritional laws as much as man; who eats with little discretion towards his health and life!

In nature there are neither rewards or punishments
– there are consequences! – Robert Ingersoll

Shorter Fasts Are Better and Safer

Here again is another reason I do not believe in long fasts unless they are carefully supervised by a health expert. The average person is not only filled with toxic poison from wrong food, air pollution, water pollution and common table salt, but they also have a residue of the many drugs they have consumed stored deep in the organs of their bodies. So a long fast to cleanse one's body might sound good in theory but, in actual practice, it is emphatically *not the case!*

In my personal experience, I have achieved greater benefits from short fasts than I have by the long fasts, even though I have supervised many long fasts. Starting with a 24 to 36 hour fast weekly, I find that the faster can really give himself a splendid internal house cleaning. The person who wishes to attain supreme vitality and agelessness can prepare for a 3 to 4 day fast by following the "No Breakfast" Plan (I regard fresh fruit as nutritional refreshment, not as a full meal) combined with a program of eating only whole, natural, organic foods for several months.

After about 4 months of the weekly fast and 4 to 6 fasts of from 3 to 4 days, a person would be ready for a 7 day fast. By this time, large amounts of toxic waste will have been removed from the body by this series of weekly and longer fasts, combined with The Bragg Healthy Lifestyle of eating healthy organic fruits, veggies and whole grains for several months. Remember, it's important to drink 8-10 glasses of distilled water daily!

With a background of 6 months of internal cleansing, the 7 day fast will prove quite simple. This first seven day fast will be a wonderful experience because the internal purification the faster experiences will be absolutely tremendous! In several more months, this person will be ready for a ten-day fast. Again this will cause a super-cleansing of every cell in the body.

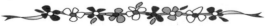

The doctor of the future will give no medicine, but will interest his patients in the care of the human frame, in diet and in the cause and prevention of disease. – Thomas A. Edison

The Faster Will Gather Marvelous Experience

Once embarked on this sensible, logical program of internal purification, you will be so imbued with the joys of your new life that fasting will become a necessary part of life itself. Day by day, while you watch the miracle of rejuvenation taking place in your body and mind, you will rejoice that you have been led to The Bragg Healthy Lifestyle of living that will make you a healthier, happier and better person every day of your life!

Why Should You Fast?

Most people spend the major part of their short lives destroying their health! But those who have found the truth have captained their lives to healthy living. It all comes down to the law of compensation. You get out of an effort just what you put into it! To me, to achieve supreme health, vitality and agelessness is worth all effort possible! I found what I want in life. I know that money cannot buy health, long life and agelessness. I follow my Bragg Healthy Lifestyle and I enjoy supreme health!

69

Every day we read about wealthy men and women who are desperately ill, many of them dying long before their time. There is no wealth that can impart or equal health and agelessness. That is the reason I often tell people that I am the richest man on earth. I am a health multibillionaire! I have the greatest wealth a person can have. I have Supreme Health 365 days of the year. I have a painless, tireless and ageless body. No one gave me my Health Wealth. I earned it by living The Bragg Healthy Lifestyle and by always staying as close to Mother Nature as possible in this polluted, poisoned world of today.

The More Often You Fast, The Longer You Will Be Able to Fast

I do not want to limit your fasting to 10 days. But I do not advise fasting any longer than 10 days until you have had, at the very least, six 10 day fasts spaced at 3 month intervals. With that experience behind you, you could graduate to a 15 day fast. By then you have done a tremendous amount of internal house cleaning.

Great Benefits From Short and Long Fasts

If you are ready to attempt a 21 or 30 day fast you know now how to conduct the fast. You now have your past fasting experience and knowledge to guide you! But, personally, I feel that my weekly 24 to 36 hour fast and my 7 to 10 day fasts 4 times a year is sufficient fasting for me. I eat only 12 meals a week and sometimes less because I never eat unless I have a genuine hunger!

Again let me state emphatically that fasting is a science. Please do not force yourself into a long fast because you think the long fast is going to do wonders, unless you are under the strict supervision of a health expert. And even the expert may decide that you would benefit more from shorter fasts to first condition yourself to a longer fast. Your 24 to 36 hour weekly fast, your 3 or 4 day fasts and your 7 to 10 day fasts will provide you with the fasting experience you will definitely need should you wish to try a longer fast later.

I have found in my research on fasting that even the health experts disagree on how long one should fast to get the very best results. Health opinions worldwide vary on fasting lengths from 7 to 30 days. I personally don't believe in the longer fast unless it is really an emergency – and then it is imperative that it be supervised by a health expert. I have thousands of students worldwide following this fasting program I'm presenting to you in this book. They are delighted and satisfied with the marvelous health benefits they enjoy!

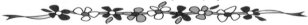

Distilled water is the greatest solvent on earth, the only water that can be taken into the body without damage to the tissues. – Dr. Allen Banik, *The Choice is Clear*

It's the song you sing and the smiles you wear, that is making the sunshine everywhere. – James Whitcomb Riley

The physician must be experienced in many things, but most assuredly in rubbing (healing massage). – Hippocrates, father of medicine

Through our actions and deeds, rather than promises, let us display the essence of love – perfect harmony in motion! – Philip Glyn, Welsh Poet

Fasting Appreciated Worldwide

The German fasting resorts believe the ideal fast is 21 days. The French are in favor of not more than a 14 day fast. In England they feel a 30 day fast is best. In our American fasting resorts, many of the fasts are supervised from 14 to 30 days.

I have found that in foreign and American fasting resorts, the directors are dedicated men and women who have a thorough knowledge of fasting. They all have been highly successful with people who have various complicated physical problems.

Fasting is a great and wonderful science and there is much to learn about it. I have been supervising fasts for over 70 years. During these years I have faithfully fasted and have enjoyed wonderful benefits! It is my honest opinion that if anyone fasts over 10 days they should be under the guidance of a health expert they can call.

I believe that the average person can fast 10 days without any complications. The 10 day fast results in a great amount of internal housecleaning. I sincerely hope I am not putting any fearful thoughts in your mind about the great science of fasting. There are thousands of people around the world who supervise their own fasts and some for even 20 or 30 days. When I speak on fasting at the Bragg Health Crusades worldwide, I ask my students how many of them have supervised their own fasts. I found that thousands of Bragg followers have fasted 20 and 30 days or more with great results!

But, I still feel that if a person is going to take a 30 day fast, it should be under the guidance of a health expert, who knows how to control long fasts. They are always ready to help you when the toxic poisons are being eliminated more heavily. They might advise you to break the fast, because they feel you may have loosened enough toxic poisons for this particular fast. Always be flexible, kind and loving to your body.

Cattle know when to go home from grazing, but a foolish man never knows his stomach's measures. – Scandinavian Proverb

Short Fasts Need Good Nutrition and Good Living Habits Between Them

I know that the wheels of progress grind slowly, but surely. Here is my theory on the science of fasting. We are dealing with human nature and there are many fears in each of us. I believe that more people will experiment with the science of fasting if they do short fasts. Many people are willing to try a 24 or a 36 hour fast and, when they find that they feel better and look better, they will then attempt a 3 day fast because they now have more confidence. The next thing you know, they will fast very successfully for 7 to 10 days. Many of my students who took several 10 day fasts had such good results that they tried a 15 day fast. Some even went on to 21 day fasts and others tried the full 30 day fast by themselves.

But they wisely started with the 24 hour fast and then graduated to the longer fast. The more experience and good results you gain, the stronger belief you will have in fasting. If you have never fasted before, start with 24 or 36 hour fast each week. I urge you to be the judge of the wonder-working miracle powers of the fast.

72

Then you may graduate to the 3 to 4 day fast and, after that, to a 7 to 10 day fast that will make you very proud of your willpower. You can accomplish a great amount of internal cleansing on short fasts. Remember, it is cumulative. The more you fast, the cleaner you become inside. Just make sure that between fasts you are living a good, healthy life!

Pre-Cleanse For Better Fasting Results

If you prepare for a fast by eating a cleansing diet for 1 to 2 days, this can greatly facilitate the cleansing process. Fresh variety salads, fresh vegetables and fruits and their juices, as well as green drinks (alfalfa, barley, chlorophyll, chlorella, spirulina, wheatgrass, etc.) stimulate waste elimination. Live, fresh foods and juices can literally pick up dead matter from your body and carry it away. Following this pre-cleansing diet you can now start your liquid fast.

Here is My Personal Fasting Program – Which I Recommend for Bragg Students

I know the great benefits I have received from fasting, and that goes for my whole family. Every week I take a 24 to 36 hour fast. I never miss this! In addition I fast from 7 to 10 days, 4 times a year.

Over the many years that I have been following this schedule, I have kept myself in superior health. I am a human dynamo! I get more living out of 1 day than most people get out of 5. I have unlimited energy for work and play! I never get tired - sleepy, yes. But never do I get that worn out, exhausted feeling. I keep myself active mentally, physically and spiritually! I maintain a heavy lecture schedule and I travel worldwide. I write and have many duties to perform. But I still make time for an enormous amount of vigorous physical activity.

All of my sports and play time is spent with youthful men and women who don't recognize calendar years and who are ageless in body, mind and spirit as I am. Otherwise, I keep far, far away from prematurely old people because most of them are so negative! Sad facts – millions have convinced themselves they are old and broken. This the reason they are ready for the scrap heap! Many of them died mentally years ago and have joined the half-alive generation.

My daughter Patricia and I belong to hiking, tennis and beach clubs, gyms, mountain climbing clubs and dancing clubs. We love ballroom dancing and South American dances like the samba, tango, etc. and fast moving steps that give us a chance to be physically active and mentally joyous. Try it – turn the music on and dance! It's fun! We enjoy doing the Hawaiian dance – the Hula. When at home in Hawaii, we enjoy giving health buffet parties along with some Hawaiian musical entertainment, singing and dancing.

When your body is cleansed by fasting and living a naturally healthy life, you will discover you feel wonderful all the time. This is because God and Mother Nature intended people to be healthy, happy and well-balanced; free of fears, frustrations, stresses and strains!

Breaking Health Laws – You Pay the Price!

I want it definitely understood that man cannot break a Natural Law. He only breaks himself while attempting to break the Natural Law. Can man break the law of gravity? Can man jump off a 25 story building and live? Of course he can't! This also applies to Mother Nature's Laws. Man has been brainwashed into eating the processed, devitalized foods which have propelled him into a pitiful physical condition. Americans are so gullible that most believe the false propaganda passed out by big "special interests," describing what healthy, long-lived people we are. **Sickness is costly big business!**

Who spends more money for doctors, nurses, hospitals, surgery, drugs and health insurance?

AMERICA DOES!

Who spends more money in the pursuit of health than any other nation in the whole, wide world?

AMERICA DOES!

Which nation has more "drives" to collect funds to fight the many diseases that plague our population?

AMERICA DOES!

Who has more convalescent homes, mental clinics and institutions than any other country in the world?

AMERICA DOES!

What nation spends the most money on magazine, newspaper, TV and radio advertising promoting "do it yourself," over-the-counter drug medication?

AMERICA DOES!

What nation takes the most sleeping pills, laxatives, aspirin and other pain killers?

AMERICA DOES!

We even have children's aspirin. Sadly, it seems they need painkillers! Aspirin in any form – be it buffered, plain or mixed with other compounds – masks the problem instead of solving it. Pain is the body's alarm.

Chapter 8

How to Break a 24 Hour Fast

Follow These Instructions Carefully!

Your 24 hour fast can be from lunch to lunch or from dinner to dinner, as long as you abstain from all solid foods. This also means no fruit or vegetable juices! This is known as the absolute distilled water fast.

One exception to the 24 hour fast is to add one teaspoon of raw honey and one teaspoon of Braggs Organic Raw Apple Cider Vinegar or fresh lemon juice to at least 3 of your 8 to 10 glasses of distilled water. This is not to help you "keep up your strength." This acts as a mucus and toxin dissolver, plus makes the water more palatable. This helps flush the debris out through the great natural filters of the body – the kidneys. They play a vital part in your fast. This is why it is important during any fast to drink 8 to 10 glasses of pure, distilled water.

I have told you how important it is to save the urine after a 24 hour fast. Just put it in a tightly sealed labeled bottle and let it settle for several weeks. You will see with your own eyes the poisons – such as mucus, salt crystals and toxins – that have been flushed out of your body by your miracle-working kidneys.

Your Kidneys – The Miracle Organs

Just think of it – each of the 2 kidneys in your body have a million efficient filters. When the body is fasting, the kidneys step up their work of detoxification. All of the Vital Force and nervous energy of the body is now working overtime to cleanse and heal your body, because it's not being used up in the laborious task of mastication, digestion, metabolism and elimination. You have no idea how powerful the Vital Force is in your body until you experience this great fasting body renovation!

The three greatest letters in the English alphabet are N-O-W.
There is no time like the present. Begin now! – Sir Walter Scott

Some Discomfort is Normal When Cleansing

Remember that as long as there is any toxic waste in your circulation, you may feel some discomfort during your fast. Soon as the Vital Force flushes these poisons out through your kidneys, you will start to feel better.

Many times during a fast, old drugs that have been buried in your system for years are loosened up and flushed out of the body. Let me tell you of one of my greatest experiences when I first started fasting. Now, let's go back to my early childhood diet. I was born and reared in Virginia and I was fed a typically greasy, starchy, fatty and sugary diet. My body was so filled with toxins as a child that I had every known childhood disease: mumps, measles, whooping cough . . . you name them and I had them! Along with these childhood miseries, I was given large amounts of a drug known as "Calomel" – and this drug was filled with quicksilver (mercury)!

A Swiss Doctor Was My Human Savior

After I was restored to a good state of health at Dr. August Rollier's Sanitarium in Leysen, Switzerland, I started my regular fasting program – which I am proud to say I have continued through all these wonderful years since then! I fasted one 24 hour period weekly and 4 times a year at 3 month intervals, I fasted from 7 to 10 days – always on a distilled water fast. After I had been on this fasting program for 5 years, it was during one of my 10 day fasts that a great miracle happened to me!

I was at my family's old homestead in Virginia. On about the seventh day of a 10 day fast, I was out in a canoe on the river leisurely enjoying the sunshine and fresh air when suddenly, without warning, I doubled up with stomach cramps. I thought I would never be able to stand the pain! With great effort I got ashore and then it happened. I had a terrific bowel evacuation! At the end of this evacuation, I felt a heavy, cool sensation in my rectum and out passed a ⅓ cup of the quicksilver from the toxic Calomel that I took in my childhood.

Healthy, organic foods have a wonderful abundance of potential life energy!

That experience marked a new day in my entire physical structure. From that day on I knew what superior health meant! My Vital Force was increased so greatly with my program of eating natural living foods, fasting, sunshine and exercise that all my body cells rejoiced with my new Energy Power! With fasting I eliminated the drugs that were given to me in my youth.

Keep Your Morale High

Please understand, even when you take a 1 day fast you are cleansing and purifying your whole body. The very thought that you are building a painless, tireless and ageless body should be an incentive to keep your morale high during your fast. Don't allow self-pity or negative thoughts to get in your mind when fasting.

Repeat these powerful affirmations when fasting:

- I have this day put my body in the hands of God and Mother Nature. I have turned to the highest power for internal purification and rejuvenation.
- Every minute that I fast I am flushing dangerous poisons that do great damage from my wonderful body. Every hour that I fast I become happier, healthier and have more energy.
- Hour by hour, my body is purifying itself.
- When I fast I am using the same method for physical, mental and spiritual purification that the greatest spiritual leaders have used throughout the ages.
- I am in complete control of my body during this fast. No false hunger pains will stop me from fasting. I will carry my fast through to a successful conclusion because I have total faith in God and Mother Nature!

Just remember, you must give instructions to all the cells of your body with your total mind and heart. The thoughts you send to your body are going to be carried out by your cells. That is the reason I urge you to not discuss your fasting program with relatives or friends. Most would give you a negative reaction. Fasting is a personal matter and please keep it that way!

77

Fasts are vitally important for they give the body a break from the digestive process, and allow it to release any stored toxins and get them out.

Keep Your Meals Healthy and Simple

When the toxins are passing out of your body and you feel some discomfort, just say to yourself . . ."This too will also pass." Be strong-minded when you fast! Think of the wonderful results you are going to achieve by fasting. Rejoice that you have been led to this great natural cleansing and rejuvenation miracle.

At the end of every fast, the very first food that reaches your taste buds should be a raw coleslaw cabbage salad – a base of chopped cabbage, grated carrots and beets. For a dressing try fresh lemon or orange squeezed over the salad. This salad acts as "nature's broom," it sweeps your intestines clean. It makes the muscles along the gastrointestinal tract work hard. If you want more have a bowl of freshly stewed (or salt-free canned) tomatoes. Stewed tomatoes are not acid-forming except when prepared with white sugar or hunks of refined, white bread. Or have a serving of delicious steamed greens – such as kale, chard, collard or beet tops with tomatoes and fresh garlic. Serve in bowls, over greens sprinkle Brewers Yeast flakes, spray Bragg Aminos, ⅓ tsp Bragg Vinegar and ⅓ tsp virgin olive oil. Try it – it's delicious! Remember, keep meals simple and natural.

Please never break a fast with animal products such as meat, milk, cheese, butter, fish or heavy nuts or seeds. After a 24 or 36 hour fast, wait until the second or third meal before you eat the heavier foods and beans, brown rice, potatoes, etc. Remember, we prefer you eat the vegetarian proteins – they are healthier! Please read the important "Foods to Avoid List," on page 237 for your not-to-buy guide when shopping.

Old age is not a time of life. It is a condition of the body. It is not time that ages the body, it is abuse that does! – Herbert Shelton

Good Health, generated by physical fitness, is the logical starting point for the pursuit of excellence in any field. Physical vitality promotes mental vitality and thus is essential to executive achievement. – Dr. Richard E. Dutton

The body and the mind are so closely connected that not even a single word or thought can come into existence without being reflected in the personality and health of the individual. – John Prentiss

The Vegetarian Diet is Healthiest!

Vegetarians are healthier and live longer! If you must eat meat and fish, please don't consume it more than 2 to 3 times weekly. Eat whole grain health breads – they are best lightly dry toasted into a melba-like toast so the starch is converted into what we call "blood sugar". See page 89 for Patricia's recipe on garlic toast. Sprinkle the large flake nutritional yeast over salads, veggies, potatoes and soups. This gives your body the B vitamins for your nervous system and also a healthier elimination.

Don't Worry About Bowels During the Fast

One of the greatest worries most people who fast have during a fast lasting from 3 to 10 days is that their bowels may stop moving. Let me emphasize that you shouldn't worry about bowel movement during a fast! This will adjust itself shortly after each fast is ended, so forget all about bowel movements and think about the wonderful purification that your body is experiencing. Mother Nature's plumbing system works perfectly if you will allow it to. When the fast is over and you eat meals that are well-balanced in bulk, moisture and lubrication, your bowels will move better than ever! You should try to eat 60% to 70% of your foods in their raw state in the form of organic salads, sprouts, fruits, veggies and fresh juices.

Living The Bragg Healthy Lifestyle will promote a healthier colon and regular elimination. You can also add 1 to 3 teaspoons of this cleansing mixture (mix ½ oat bran and ½ psyllium husk powder) to your liquids and foods 2 to 3 times daily. This mixture works wonders!

Another miracle to try are flax seeds. I introduced them years ago and millions have benefitted. Soak 3 tbsps of flax seeds in cup of distilled water for 3 hours (gets gel-like). Add 1 tbsp to cup of water and drink an hour after dinner. You can presoak enough mixture for 2 to 3 days and keep in fridge. Use as a hot or cold drink, add honey if desired. It's not only good for elimination, but flax seeds are rich in omega-3 for your heart.

Almost every human malady is connected, either by highway or byway, with the stomach. – Sir Francis Head

We Seldom Recommend Enemas or Colonics

For easier-flowing bowel movements:
Squatting is the natural way to have a
bowel movement. It opens up the anal
area more directly. When on the toilet,
putting your feet up 6 to 8 inches on a
waste basket or footstool gives you the
same squatting effect. From behind use
two fingers to gently pull up on the edge
of the anus – this helps it roll out easier!

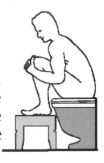

Some books on fasting recommend that you should
have an enema or colonic daily during a fast. I want it
understood that I feel enemas and colonics during fasts
are usually unnecessary. The only time I would suggest
them is during extreme constipation, in an emergency
or on the advice of your health practitioner. When the
bowel refuses to evacuate, or in illness, extreme gas or
bloating, an enema of warm, distilled water with 3 Tbsp
of fresh lemon or aloe juice is strictly a temporary means
to get bowels cleansed and moving.

In comparing the enema to a powerful laxative, we
would say that the enema is superior to the drug laxative
– but it certainly has its own faults. If you continue to
use enemas, laxatives or colonics over a long period of
time, it will irritate your bowel and wash out important
internal secretions (healthy intestinal flora or *"friendly
bacteria"*) necessary for good bowel function. To replace
the flora lost due to antibiotics, drugs, yeast infections,
candidiasis or colon abuse, a 40 to 60 minute retention
enema can be helpful. Use warm, distilled water with 1
to 2 teaspoons of acidophilus powder or liquid added.

During a fast, your body is having a rest! Since no
food is being eaten, there might be only 1 or 2 or even
no bowel movements during the fast. Your elimination
system is having a rest. It's best not to disturb it. The
body has its own sanitation and antiseptic system within
the bowel. Don't worry, in most situations you don't
need enemas. When you have finished your fast and
begin eating raw, healthy foods and living The Bragg
Healthy Lifestyle, your eliminations will be more regular.

Chapter 9

I Fast 7 to 10 Days, 4 Times a Year

Here's the Path to Perfect Health!

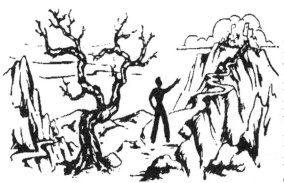

My daughter Patricia and I are very sincere and faithful to our fasting program. We know what it has done for us, for the members of our family, for our friends and for millions of Bragg health-conscious students around the world.

Our Bragg fasting program calls for 4 longer fasts a year, along with a weekly 24 to 36 hour fast. Fasting helps cleanse and keep your body healthy. These cleansing fasts will help you live a longer, healthier and more vital life! So, my calendar calls for an early January fast. Sometimes this fast only lasts 7 days, it may run 8 days, it may run 9 days, and it may extend the full 10 days.

At the beginning of each year I mark the days that I am going to fast for 7 to 10 days. You may wonder why I say 7 to 10 days. Sometimes I fast only 7 days because I feel that in that time I have accomplished the necessary house cleaning of my body. Be flexible on dates if you feel a cold coming on. Colds call for an earlier start to your fast to help cleanse out the mucus toxins. Colds indicate your body needs detoxifying and a good cleansing. A cold is Mother Nature forcing you to fast!

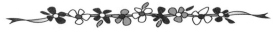

Hippocrates, Aristotle, Galen, Paracelsus, Plato, Socrates and other great philosophers, scientists and physicians for centuries have used fasting as a method of cleansing, healing and renewing the body.

81

Fasting Balances Your Thermostat Naturally

I have fasted for so many years that I am perceptive to what a fast is doing for me. My inner voice seems to tell me when it's time to break each fast. Remember, let your body and inner voice guide you – for your body wants you healthy and alive and the toxins removed!

I always mark on my calendar a fast for my spring "house cleaning." My spring fast always runs the full 10 days because that is when I truly want to clean house after a long winter. During our Bragg Health Crusades, I am often forced to talk in over-heated halls and auditoriums. I am sorry to say that most humans cannot take the cold weather, nor can they stand a fresh, healthy, well-ventilated hall. So I must forget my feelings and lecture in these over-heated halls to the hot-house plants of modern civilization that most people have become.

Fasting so greatly purifies the body and so exhilarates the body's functions that the thermostatic system of the body works with more efficiency. For instance, I can leave my desert home near Palm Springs, California, in January – when the heat averages in the 80s during the day and the nights in the 60s – board an airplane to Midwestern cities such as Duluth or Minneapolis, Minnesota or to a Canadian city such as Toronto – where the temperature will be as low as 10 to 30 degrees below zero and, because of fasting and natural living, my body will adjust easily to this bitterly cold weather.

I find I can take the most frigid weather better than most of the inhabitants who are supposedly acclimated to their own climate. This ability to adjust to climate is only one of the many fasting miracles that happen to the body. Fasting gives the body a chance to flush out the toxic poisons and build up its Vital Force.

But, as I have stated earlier, when I go to the cities that are locked in freezing weather, I find that their halls and auditoriums are overheated. There is so little oxygen in the air that my body will naturally absorb some of the carbon dioxide that people expel from their lungs during the breathing process. That is why my spring fasting is so valuable. I want that 10 day fast to flush out of my body any accumulated toxins, plus any other toxic poisons that are found in those artificially heated rooms. That's why my springtime fast is always 7 to 10 days.

Then when summer rolls around, I take a 7 day fast in late July or August. This is the easiest of all my fasts because I have been eating large amounts of luscious, fresh fruits and garden-fresh organically grown vegetables. I believe I enjoy my summer fast more than any other. In fact, this fast is so easy that I never stop either my heavy physical exercise or mental activities. My autumn fast can be anytime in late October or during November. It also extends from 7 to 10 days.

Fasting truly has many cumulative miracle effects. I fast about 75 days a year. It's a great physiological rest I give my digestive organs. This includes my liver, gallbladder, and all the other faithful organs, including the ones producing hormones, that are running my body and keeping me healthy! The physiological rest that I give my pancreas allows it to produce ample insulin. This also goes for the stomach, where so many digestive juices are needed to handle all my food intake.

Mother Nature Intended the Body and Breath to Be Sweet and Free from Odors

You will find after a fast that you'll have more saliva which contains the important enzyme amylase. You will discover that your mouth will taste sweeter and your breath will be clean. The more you fast, the less mouth and body odor you will have! I never need deodorants.

Several years ago I supervised a fasting program for a student who came to California from New York. His problem was a terrifically bad body odor that exuded from every part of his body, particularly from under his arms, the palms of his hands and his feet. The odor can only be described as putrid. It wasn't that the man didn't take baths – because he told me that he took as many as

Health is the most natural thing in the world. It is natural to be healthy because we are a part of nature – we are nature. Nature is trying hard to keep us well, because she needs us in her business. – Elbert Hubbard

3 and 4 hot, soapy showers or baths daily and would use all kinds of deodorants or antiperspirants. But it was all to no avail, for that horrible odor persisted. He was becoming a nervous wreck because he felt like a social outcast. He not only had a bad body odor, but he had such heavy halitosis his breath could knock you over! He used gargles, lozenges, chewed mint gum, but still that rancid, bad breath persisted.

Unhealthy Lifestyle Causes Chronic Fatigue

When questioning this man before putting him on his first fast, I found that he had been enervated by terrible lifestyle habits, overwork, marital difficulties and heavy financial responsibilities. When you enervate yourself, over-expend your nervous energy and exhaust your Vital Force, the organs of elimination cannot do their job effectively and efficiently. This man was plainly suffering from nerve chronic fatigue! His eating habits were unhealthy. His working day was so busy that he would gobble a sandwich and wash it down with coffee. He simply didn't take time to prepare healthy meals. He was constipated and his elimination was off it's rhythm.

I told him it had taken years to get his body into this decaying condition and that a program of fasting and natural living would take time to accomplish its mission. But he was an intelligent and logically thinking man who fully cooperated with our Bragg Healthy Lifestyle Program. I started him on a series of 36 hour fasts and between the fasts, I gradually added more raw fruit and vegetables to his heavily concentrated diet of refined sugars, fats and meat. I believe there must be a transition period between changing from a unhealthy diet to a healthy diet. It's best not to force the body to change quickly. You must take things slowly. Instead of eating meat 3 times a day, he now ate meat only once a day. He had been a great eater of white bread, so I substituted 100% whole grain breads. It's best oven dry toasted.

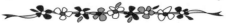

Use your feet as Mother Nature intended. Give them every possible freedom. Go barefoot every chance you get. I do! For more info read our Foot Book!
– Patricia Bragg

Fasting Pulls Out Toxins and Poisons

In time I put him on a 7 day fast. The first three days were rough because he was now eliminating large amounts of toxic poisons. He vomited some mucus and yellowish-green bile during the first 4 days and on the 5th day he broke out in a cleansing rash that lasted a few days, then vanished. The odor that came from his body and breath was almost unbearable! He gave me a specimen of his first urine every morning. He sealed it tightly, dated it and stored it on a shelf to settle. Be sure and do this. Fasting is a cleansing-healing miracle! The proof is the foul urine that comes out!

I am well-acquainted with the sickening odor of putrid urine, being a health practitioner and a Physical Therapist. In my many years in the health field, I've spent time in hospitals and health spas inspiring patients to cleanse; recover their health; be strong; always live a healthy lifestyle; and treasure and protect their life!

After his 7 day fast, I eliminated more refined foods and gave him more raw fruits and vegetables. After several more weeks, I put him on a 10 day fast. This was a much easier fast for him, but he still eliminated heavy amounts of toxic matter. This is called the "latent poison" that becomes concentrated in the cells of the body. It takes time with regular fasting and an alkaline-rich diet of fresh fruits and salads to slowly dislodge these deeply stored, deadly toxins and poisons.

Often people will say to me, "Well, with all due respect to your philosophy of living, I am a perfectly healthy person. I eat what agrees with me, drink all the coffee I want and eat what normal people eat." But I know better, I know poisons are accumulating in their tissues. I know some day it will break loose and they will become deathly ill with a variety of illnesses – aches, pains, headaches, colds, flu, rashes, etc. – as this healing crisis is trying to clean out the toxins. That's what disease and sickness are – Mother Nature trying to cleanse and purify the burdened body of toxins, accumulated since childhood, by pushing these toxins out!

Many people aim to do right, but are just poor shots.

You Pay For Your Sins Sooner or Later

Many people inherit constitutions of steel through heredity. They can laugh and flaunt at God and Mother Nature's Laws and seem to get away with it! Inevitably the day of reckoning always arrives, the day when Mother Nature starts a purification by some form of elimination. I have seen so-called healthy people who thought they could eat and drink anything, smoke, lose sleep and work long hours – suddenly collapse with a heart attack, stroke or illness. Sadly, I have seen many of these powerful people go to an early grave due to their disregard of common sense health laws!

So I knew that my student had to be handled very carefully. It pleased me that he kept up his program persistently and faithfully. It took almost a year of weekly 24 to 36 hour fasts and strong adherence to The Bragg Healthy Lifestyle to defeat his annoying body odors. Today that man has a sweet, clean breath. There is no longer any putrid odor exuding from his body. He is an entirely different man. He not only defeated the enemies within his body, but he looks and feels 20 years younger. He's now handsome, youthful and vigorous, with personal magnetism. He's more relaxed because he has a healthy body and a healthy, peaceful mind. Now it must be very plain and obvious to you why I use fasting as an effective, safe method of detoxifying the body. Most people wait until something happens to their health before they take action – and sadly it's often too late!

An Ounce of Prevention Is Worth a Ton of Cures!

Those of you who are reading this book should not wait until Mother Nature shocks you into detoxification. Isn't it far more logical and sensible to give your body a physiological rest every week for 24 to 36 hours? Isn't it good, sound reasoning for you to take a 7 to 10 day fast from time to time and give your body a chance to purify itself? Give your body a chance to get rid of any accumulated toxins! In our modern, complex civilization we are absolutely bound to pick up poisons and toxins.

No man can violate Nature's Laws and escape her penalties! – Julian Johnson

Fasting Promotes Healthy Elimination

I have explained to you very thoroughly that this is a world filled with toxins and poisons. Our only salvation is to be faithful with a regular program of fasting. This fasting strongly promotes a healthier colon and elimination. It helps keep the body cleaner and healthier by regular purging out the vicious toxins. It can mean a whole new, cleaner life, because when you are healthy, you have more joy, peace and energy in your life.

A Normal Colon and Sick Colons

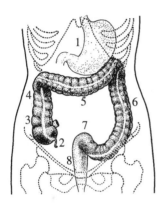

A. The Normal Colon
Proper position in relation to organs:
1) stomach 2) appendix 3) cecum
4) ascending colon 5) transverse colon
6) descending colon 7) sigmoid flexure
8) rectum

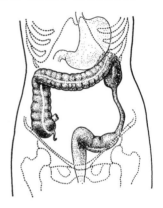

B. The Spastic Colon
Colon in spastic constipation.

87

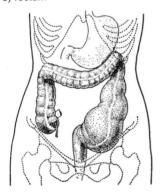

C. The Engorged Colon
Colon in engorged constipation.

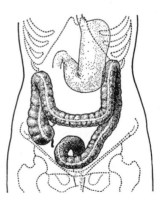

D. The Sagging Colon
Ptosis, or sagging, of transverse colon, accompanied by displacement of stomach.

What a person eats and drinks becomes his own body chemistry.

How to Conduct a 3 Day, 7 Day & 10 Day Fast

A fast of 3 days or longer should be conducted under ideal conditions. You should be able to rest any time you feel the toxins passing out of your body. During this time you might feel some discomfort. You should rest and relax quietly until the poisons have passed out of your body. It's best to be at peace and alone when possible. This brief period of discomfort will leave as soon as the loosened toxins have passed out through your kidneys, lungs, skin, etc.

During longer fasts don't tell others you're fasting. Why not? During a fast you must keep in mind only positive thoughts of the cleansing and the renewing miracles happening in your body. Often others are ignorant and uninformed about fasting and project negative thoughts.

Our fasting is such a very personal and quiet time that many years ago I went into the Santa Monica Mountains in California and bought a tract of land in the wilderness of the Topanga Canyon near Malibu. There I built a retreat cabin, identical to Thoreau's at Walden Pond. In that natural seclusion, Patricia and I enjoy the quiet and peace for our fasting time. If it's possible for you to get away to some secluded place and do your fast in Mother Nature's splendor with fresh air and solitude, you will enjoy better results!

There are also some very fine health spas throughout the world where all the conditions are perfect for a restful fast. Inquire at health stores for any located in your area. Many of the Bragg students who fast regularly tell us that they use their vacation as a period of fasting and purification of body, mind and soul. Often they will go to some beautiful spot to rent accommodations and take their fast in seclusion. I am not saying it's necessary to go away to fast. Your home is your castle and hopefully you will be cozy and peaceful there. The Bragg family all regularly fast. When any one is fasting, we have great consideration for them. We have an agreement not to ask each other how we feel during the fast. Fasting is so personal that no one can do anything for you during the fast, so it's best not to discuss it with others. Relax and be thankful for your miracle cleansing.

When you are on a fast of 3 days or more, you are really on Mother Nature's miracle operating table.

Nature is ridding you of the waste, mucus, toxins and other foreign substances in your body.

Chapter 10

How to Break Long Fasts

How to Break a 7 Day Fast

Remember that when you have been on a 7 day fast your stomach and the 30 feet of intestinal tract have contracted. When you are ready to break the fast, it should be done as follows:

Around 5 to 6 pm at the end of your 7 day fast peel and cut up 4 or 5 organic tomatoes, add ½ cup distilled water, garlic if you wish, bring them to a boil and then turn off the heat. When they are cool enough to eat, serve in bowl with the liquid and eat with a spoon. Spray some Bragg Aminos over the top and a dash of Bragg vinegar and virgin olive oil. Eat as much as you desire. On the morning of the 8th day, you are to have a salad of chopped cabbage and grated beets and carrots, with half an orange or lemon squeezed over it. After your salad, you may have a bowl of steamed greens (kale, Swiss chard, collard, mustard or beet greens) and peeled tomatoes. Bring the greens to a boil, then turn off heat. With your greens, you may eat 2 slices of 100% whole grain bread that's been oven dry toasted into a melba toast. See recipe in next paragraph for delicious garlic toast. This food should be eaten in the morning. During the day you may have all the distilled water you wish.

For dinner you may have another salad of grated cabbage, carrots, chopped celery and avocado, with fresh orange or lemon juice for dressing. Often you may not require or desire any more food. But, if so, you may have 2 to 3 cooked vegetables; such as broccoli, stringbeans, carrots, peas, okra, squash, etc. You may also have 1 to 2 pieces of whole grain garlic toast. Lightly toast slices of whole grain bread in oven. Rub raw garlic cloves on both sides of toast. Spread with olive oil and sprinkle with Bragg Liquid Aminos and large nutritional yeast flakes.

89

Prayer is the mortar that holds our house together. – Sister Teresa

On the morning of the 9th day, you may have a variety of fresh organic fruits such as banana, pineapple, papaya, grapes, orange, grapefruit and apples. Or you may have a Bragg Pep Drink, page 230. At noon you may have a salad of grated carrots, cabbage and celery and some garlic toast. At dinner you may have the Bragg Health Salad and, if desired, steamed veggies or soup.

How to Break a 10 Day Fast

There is little difference between the 7 and the 10 day fast. On the 10th day around dinner time you will have stewed tomatoes; from then you will follow the same schedule as given in the 7 day fast.

IMPORTANT – NEVER OVEREAT!

Don't eat more than you need or desire! Remember that you have been without food for 7 to 10 days. By this time, you have lost the strong craving for food. Because you eat, does not mean that you are going to immediately feel a surge of energy. It takes the body time to adjust from a detoxifying mode to eating again.

Remember – Don't Worry About Evacuation

It may take the body a day or two to adjust to eating again, so don't be concerned if your bowels are sluggish. In many instances some people will have a bowel evacuation shortly after eating their first meal after a fast. Elimination is different for each person, so we cannot set a standard when the bowels will move. I urge you to be patient with Mother Nature and don't try to force your bowels to move. Mother Nature has given the bowels their own sanitation and antiseptic system. This system will promote natural bowel movements. You are now eating healthy foods that stimulate the peristaltic or wavelike motion of the bowels. When they do begin evacuation, if you follow our instructions and always eat healthy foods, you will establish healthy regular eliminations that will naturally flush the toxins and waste matter from your body.

Behind every successful person is themselves. – New American Proverb

The Ideal Elimination Program

In my own life, by living on a diet which is rich in bulk, moisture, water and lubrication, I have established the following elimination habits. I have a bowel movement shortly after arising. I encourage this by a few waist twists and leg kicks (pg. 118) to help give me a good elimination. I told you, I don't eat breakfast because I believe the No Breakfast Plan is healthier. Several hours after arising I eat delicious organic fresh fruits or a dish of fresh fruits – sliced pineapple, bananas, oranges, etc., or the Bragg Pep Drink or a dish of prunes or sun dried apricots soaked in pineapple juice. At noon I have my first real meal of the day, usually the Bragg Raw Vegetable Salad page 231. I often add avocado to my salad – veggies and avocados are excellent lubricants in promoting healthy elimination for the gastrointestinal tract.

I make it a hard and fast rule to always eat my salad first. I do this for several reasons. First I think we must educate our 260 taste buds to accept only natural foods. Therefore when you have raw foods, either a raw vegetable salad or a fruit salad to start the meal, you educate your taste buds to enjoy and want clean, live, healthy foods.

Most people start a meal with a broth or soup with sandwiches or bread. This is wrong in my opinion! To make the taste buds keen, sharp and alive – having your raw salad or fruits at the beginning of the meal starts the digestive juices flowing for raw foods are rich in natural enzymes. All this contributes to good nutrition. I urge you to always eat something raw at the beginning of each meal. You will find in time your taste buds will begin to reject devitalized, unhealthy foods that you may be tempted to eat. As you re-educate the taste buds to enjoy more fruits and salads, you will find that you can and should increase the daily amount of raw, live foods you eat to 60% to 70% of your total intake – it's the healthiest!

You can do more for your own health and well-being than any doctor, any hospital, any drug and any exotic medical device. – Joseph Califano

The Bragg Healthy Lifestyle
Promotes Super Health & Longevity

Remember that raw foods are the live, vital foods. They are as Mother Nature made them. They're whole, natural, live foods – vibrating with enzymes and solar energy! Most people want food that stimulates them – the sugars, fats, salt, heavy, overcooked and refined foods that have little food value. They want fast foods and most of them have been stripped of their goodness.

I am not telling you to eat a 100% raw food diet, because I don't think modern people can live as their ancestors did 5 or 6 thousand years ago.

The Bragg Healthy Lifestyle consists of eating a diet of 60% to 70% fresh, live, organically grown foods; raw vegetables, salads, fresh fruits and juices; sprouts, raw seeds and nuts; all-natural 100% whole grained breads, pastas, cereals and nutritious beans and legumes. These are the no cholesterol, no fat, no salt, "live foods" that produce the body fuel that helps produce healthy, lively people. Healthy "live foods" and fasting are the main reasons people become revitalized and reborn into a fresh new life filled with youthfulness, health, vitality, joy and longevity! There are millions of healthy Bragg followers worldwide proving this lifestyle works miracles!

Vegetarianism Versus Meat Eating

Over the long years that I have been a Nutritionist, the controversy of "Vegetarianism versus Meat Eating" has raged furiously. Both sides present the most scientific reasons for their side of the story. I am not going to try to persuade you to be either a vegetarian or a meat eater. There are hundreds of books written on both subjects.

Love is the cement that binds families together, but it is friendship that makes them happy. – William Hazlitt

A wise man should consider that health is the greatest of human blessings. – Hippocrates

I enjoy eating raw vegetable salads and plenty of fresh fruit. I love natural whole grains, beans, brown rice and lentils. – Jack LaLanne

I Prefer the Healthier Vegetarian Diet

Over the years of following a program of fasting and eating a diet containing an abundance of raw organic fruit and vegetables, my body has become so keen that it practically tells me what to eat at every meal. After years on this healthy vegetarian diet, my body has lost the desire for meat, fowl and fish. My diet is composed of organic raw fruits and vegetables, cooked vegetables, beans, legumes, brown rice, etc. with raw nuts and seeds and their butters, raw wheat germ and Brewer's yeast.

This is what my body seems to thrive on. But occasionally there were times when my body told me to eat a piece of meat or a piece of fish, or to have some natural cheese or a few fertile eggs. In other words, my body developed an instinct for the selection of foods. Sometimes I go 4 or 5 years without tasting eggs, etc., then my body will telegraph that I need some. Listening to my inner voice has helped me enormously.

Basically I have been a vegetarian by nature most of my life. I was reared on a large farm in Virginia where hundreds of hogs and cattle were slaughtered regularly, so killing has always been repulsive to me. I have never been a hunter or a fisherman because I do not like to take another life. I have made 13 expeditions to distant lands and I have found many robust, healthy people living on a vegetarian diet. On the other hand, I have found people in other cultures who also enjoyed higher health and yet included animal products in their diets. I roamed the South Seas for over a year at one time and in those far flung islands I found supermen and wonder women. They not only lived on an abundance of fresh fruit and vegetables, but they included fish, fowl and some meat in their diet.

So you see I have tried to be as fair as I could about this question of Vegetarianism versus Meat Eating. I feel that as we cleanse and purify our bodies we develop a keen sense of what is healthiest and best for us to eat.

93

Nutrition directly affects growth, development, reproduction, well-being and an individual's physical and mental condition. Health depends upon nutrition more than on any other single factor. – Dr. Wm. H. Sebrell, Jr.

Eliminating Meat is Safer and Healthier

Most uninformed nutritionists call meat the #1 source of protein. Those proteins coming from the vegetable kingdom are referred to as the #2 proteins. This is a sad and terrible mistake. It should be the other way around!

In this day and age, almost all meat is laden with herbicides, fungicides, pesticides and other chemicals that are sprayed on or poured into the feed which these animals consume. They are also pumped full of hormones, antibiotics, growth stimulators and all kinds of drugs to fatten them up and keep them from dying from the extremely unhealthy conditions most of them live in! This is not to mention the admitted fact that many of them are fed the dead, ground up carcasses of other feed lot animals who, for a variety of reasons, didn't make it to the slaughterhouse.

94

Speaking of the slaughterhouse, what kind of chemical reaction do you suppose would occur in your body if somebody put a choke chain around your neck to keep you in line, shoved you onto a conveyor belt, and made you watch in horror as all of those in line in front of you were beheaded one by one? Well, your body would be pumped so full of adrenaline from all that fear you wouldn't know what hit you! Unused adrenaline is extremely toxic. If you think for a minute that most of the meat that you consume is not packed with this toxic substance, you're sadly mistaken!

Also, consider the fact that cattle, sheep, chickens, etc., are all vegetarians. When you eat them, you are just eating polluted vegetables. Why not skip all the waste and toxins and just eat healthy, organic vegetables?

And what about that myth that you have to eat meat to get your protein? If that were true, where do you suppose farm animals, especially horses, get their protein? They are vegetarians! They get their protein from the grains and grasses that they eat. You are no different. You can get the proteins you need from the large variety of whole grains, tofu, raw nuts, seeds, beans, fruits and vegetables that God put on this planet for your health. See Vegetable Protein % Chart, page 233.

Meat Has Toxic Uric Acid & Cholesterol

Meat is a major source of toxic uric acid and cholesterol, both harmful to your health. If you insist on eating meat, it should be an organically fed source and not eaten more than 2 to 3 times weekly. Fresh fish can be the least toxic of the flesh proteins, but beware of fish from polluted waters. They can be loaded with mercury, lead, cadmium, DDT and other toxic substances. If you are unsure of the waters the fish come from, don't risk eating it. Avoid shellfish – shrimp, lobster and crayfish. They are garbage-eating bottom-feeders (the rats and flies of the water world). They eat decaying scum and refuse off the bottoms of the oceans, lakes and rivers. Chickens and turkeys are a sick bunch and commercially mass fed and heavily drugged with antibiotics and hormones. Be selective and cautious in your eating; seek only the healthiest food choices.

People should not eat pork or pork products. The pig is the only animal besides man that develops arteriosclerosis. This animal is so loaded with cholesterol that in cold weather, unprotected pigs will become stiff, as though frozen solid. Pigs are often infected with a dangerous parasite which causes the disease trichinosis.

Patricia and I enjoy being vegetarians and not polluting our bodies with unhealthy meat, fowl and fish proteins. It's safer and healthier getting our proteins from organic vegetables, beans, legumes, nuts, etc. Please refer often to the Vegetable Protein % Chart, page 233.

Seven of My Beloved Teachers

One of the greatest teachers and physicians in the science of body purification and nutrition was Dr. John Tilden, M.D., of Denver. This great scientist will surely go down in history as one of the finest physicians. His program included fasting and an abundance of fresh fruits and vegetables. He lived into his 90s and was active to the end of his life keeping his patients healthy.

Another of the finest doctors who specialized in nutrition was the famed Dr. John Harvey Kellogg, M.D. He was the director for 60 years of the famous Battle Creek Sanitarium in Battle Creek, Michigan.

Dedicated Great Health Healers

Dr. Kellogg's sanitarium specialized in a vegetarian diet and people from around the world were restored to radiant health by following his health program. I had the privilege of studying under Dr. Kellogg and it was one of the outstanding experiences of my early career.

In my early career, I was associated with Bernarr Macfadden, the Father and Founder of the Physical Culture Movement. Macfadden tried vegetarianism for a time, but gradually went back to a mixed diet which included meat and fish. He lived healthy and active to nearly 88 years of age and he believed in mixing proteins.

Over my many years in the health field, I have met many famous men and women who restored thousands of people to health through natural methods. In the 1920s I worked with Dr. St. Louis Estes, D.D.S., who was a pioneer and strict believer in the raw food diet. I saw many broken, weak, sick people restored to health by changing to his raw food diet. (I feel it's best to have a healthy balance of 60% to 70% raw foods. – P.B.)

Dr. Benedict Lust, M.D., was the Father and Founder of Naturopathy in America. He established in New York a great school of Naturopathy which educated and graduated hundreds of Naturopathic Doctors who have used and spread his teachings around the world.

Dr. Henry Lindlahr, M.D., was a famous drugless physician who lobbied for the return to natural methods in the modern treatment and prevention of disease.

Professor Arnold Ehret was one of the world's greatest food scientists. He was the discoverer and creator of "The Mucusless Diet Healing System," which is a strictly vegetarian regime. I know many of Professor Ehret's students who are in their 80s and 90s and still enjoy vigorous, robust health by following his vegetarian plan.

Fasting Credo of the famous Buchinger Clinics in Germany and Spain:
We must restore fasting to the place it occupied in an ancient hierarchy of values "above medicine." We must rediscover it and restore it to honor because it is a necessity. A beneficial fast of several weeks, as practised in the earliest days of the Church, was to give strength, life and health to the body and soul of all Christians who had the faith and courage to practice fasting.

Chapter 11

Your Tongue Never Lies – It's Your Inside Magic Mirror

Your tongue – your inside magic mirror – reveals how much toxic material is stored in the cells and vital organs of your body. The tongue is the mirror of the stomach and of the entire membrane system.

In your body there is a hose-like tube that averages 30 feet long, extending from the mouth to the anus. It has the body heat of 98.6°, plus body moisture. Through this tube passes all the food you eat. Now, different foods take different times to pass through the tube. Sad facts – most people eat an unhealthy, refined, concentrated, acid-forming diet. They eat large amounts of refined white flour, white sugar, salt and saturated fats. Most of these commercial foods lack sufficient bulk, moisture and lubrication to pass quickly through the 30 foot tube.

I believe that there is a common factor that precedes or is coexistent with most body ills that afflict us. This common denominator is constipation. Definitions may differ but it is logical that if outgo does not equal intake – either in terms of quantity or in frequency – then constipation will occur and it can be the beginning of more serious physical problems.

Most people are brainwashed to believe there is no harm in eating almost anything, as often as they desire it. We are told to eat big breakfasts to furnish plenty of energy to last all morning. Soon after breakfast they consume more food, donuts, etc. at mid-morning coffee breaks. Then comes lunch, then a mid-afternoon coffee break followed by the usual heavy evening meal, later TV snacks and a bedtime snack before retiring. On top of all this food, many people will gorge on snacks of candy, salted nuts, cakes, pies, cookies and ice cream, etc. This means that food is ingested six or more times a day, literally stuffing and overworking your stomach!

The Body Can Take a Lot of Abuse!

The average person believes that if they have one good bowel movement a day, usually in the morning, that they are free of constipation. One full bowel movement is not sufficient to remove all of the food material these people are stuffing into their intestinal tracts. As a consequence this rotten, putrefying, morbid waste lies undischarged in the intestine, where it undergoes enzymatic and bacteriological changes that often cause severe physical problems.

The human body is basically strong and can take a lot of abuse from over-stuffing, plus eating unhealthy meals. It is most difficult to tell these people who eat incorrectly and have only one bowel movement a day that they are constipated and thus are inviting serious troubles later. But there is one warning signal – an unhealthy tongue – that can tell these people that they are carrying a nasty cesspool within their bodies.

If these people fasted for 2 or 3 days on distilled water exclusively, their "Magic Mirror" tongue would tell them quite plainly that they are carrying a horrible mass of fermenting poison inside of their intestines. A few days of fasting will coat the tongue with a thick, white, toxic material that has a strong odor. This heavy coating can be scraped off and examined. In fact, you can scrape the tongue clean but, in a few hours, the toxic coating usually returns. This is an indication of the amount of putrefying toxic filth, mucus and other poisons that are accumulated in the body's cells that are now being eliminated from the inside surface of the stomach, intestines, organs and from all parts the body.

The actual amount of toxic material the average person carries around with them is almost unbelievable! In my opinion, many physical problems are the result of this clogging of the 30 foot intestinal tube, the circulation, cells and the entire pipe system of the human body. I believe that these poisons cause a constitutional clogging of the entire human pipe system, especially plugging up the microscopically tiny capillaries.

Learn to Read Your Tongue's Message

Mother Nature shows the faster by coating the tongue that his body contains toxic poisons. The characteristics of tissue construction especially of the powerful, vital internal organs – such as the kidneys, liver and all the glands – are like those of a sponge. Imagine a sponge filled with a putrefying mass of thick paste. I have supervised thousands of fasts and only a person with my long experience knows the great amount of toxins that are stored in the body of the average person who is trying to survive on the standard American diet.

Think of a simple illustration for instance, someone with a common cold. Have you ever stopped to think how much mucus and phlegm passes out of the body through the nose and throat? This is also how the vital organs such as the lungs, kidneys and bladder are passing out poisons during this cleansing crisis.

So start right now to learn more about yourself by fasting and closely watching your tongue. The tongue is a spongy organ whose surface accurately mirrors the health or ill health of every other part of your body. The "Magic Mirror" can be a guiding star in your journey to Super Health. The more faithfully you follow a good fasting schedule and the more accurately you follow a program of natural eating, the cleaner your tongue will become during a fast.

This is a definite signpost that you are on the New Life Road – a life free of physical problems and misery. This road will lead to your greatest achievement – an Ageless, Painless and Tireless Body! So, as you go on your 24 to 36 hour or 7 to 10 day fast, note how much cleaner your tongue becomes with each fast. This will reveal the amazing *Miracles of Fasting* to you.

A fast can help you heal with greater speed; cleanse your liver, kidneys and colon; purify your blood; help you lose excess weight and water; flush out toxins; clear the eyes and tongue, and cleanse the breath.
– James F. Balch, M.D. *Prescription for Nutritional Healing*

Open your mind, for the doors of wisdom are never shut. – Ben Franklin

Man does not die of old age! It's been proven there are no special diseases due simply to old age. Most diseases kill both young and old. Many diseases start from a body loaded with toxic poisons. Keep the body clean by following your regular fasting program plus eating only healthy foods. Your tongue and urine can be your guideposts to internal purity. Watch both carefully with respect when you do a cleansing fast.

TIME

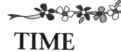

I have just a little minute,
Only sixty seconds in it,
Just a tiny little minute,
Give account if I abuse it;
Forced upon me; can't refuse it.
Didn't seek it, didn't choose it.
But it's up to me to use it.
I must suffer if I lose it;
But eternity is in it.
  – Unknown

100

Pure Water (H_2O) is Essential for Health

Pure, distilled water is the best for your health.
It's free of inorganic minerals and harmful chemicals.

Read the Bragg Book, *Water – The Shocking Truth*.
See back pages for booklist.

To maintain good health, the body must be exercised properly (stretching, walking, jogging, running, biking, swimming, deep breathing, good posture, etc.) and nourished wisely (natural foods), so to maintain a normal weight and increase the good life of radiant health, peace, joy and happiness. – Paul C. Bragg

---

Dream big, think big, but enjoy the small
miracles of daily life! – Patricia Bragg

If you truly love Nature, you will find Beauty everywhere.
  – Vincent Van Gogh

Earth laughs and smiles in flowers. – Ralph Waldo Emerson

Chapter 12

Just Grin and Bear It

"I want to fast because I believe it would do wonders for me, but how can I fast and yet escape the great feeling of hunger that the first 3 days of fasting produces?" That is the question that is put to us many, many times when I discuss the Miracle of Fasting at our Bragg Health Crusade lectures all over the world. We can give only one answer "Just Grin and Bear It."

"I tried a fast once, but I got weak and felt miserable, I just had to start eating." We often hear this line.

Nowhere in this book have I stated that fasting is easy. Eating regularly has become such an ingrained part of people's lives that, if you take food away from them, they experience many mental and physical reactions. That is the very reason why fasting is not popular. Humans are creatures of strong habits. Most people automatically eat 3 or more meals every day and not because they have earned their food with physical activity. They have been brainwashed to believe everyone should eat at certain hours for regular mealtimes.

Patricia and I had the pleasure of staying at the fabulous Mauna Kea Hotel, on the Island of Hawaii. It's an American-plan hotel, which means the cost per day for your room includes meals. Breakfast started at 7:30 am, luncheon began at 12:30 pm and dinner at 7 pm. We passed the dining room at these hours, the guests were all eagerly waiting for the doors to open so they could get at the expansive buffet.

Were they hungry at exactly these hours? How could they be? Most of the guests did nothing but relax on the beach, socialize, drive golf carts, play cards or read!

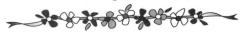

*It is a mistake to think that the more a man eats,
the stronger he will become.*

Don't Live to Eat – Eat to Live & Be Healthy

The hotel guests did absolutely nothing to earn all these meals, but they paid for them and felt they should eat them. The same thing happens on cruise ships. There is always a crowd waiting for the dining room to open so they can eat what they paid for.

Food! It can be a blessing to man, but also a curse! The human body can take a lot of abuse from overfeeding. But there comes a day when the body's digestive system becomes over-stuffed, overworked and overwhelmed, it's then that health problems begin.

Digestive troubles plague modern man. Constipation heads the list of his miseries. Tons upon tons of pills, powders and liquids are sold to try and flush out the waste packed into people's intestines and colon. Modern man packs food into himself faster than the functions of digestion and elimination can handle it. This is very much like trying to race your car with the brakes on.

102

There is scientific reasoning that constipation is the foundation of many other body ailments. The reasoning behind this conclusion is sound. If constipation means retention of waste, here's a simple test you can take. Prepare your next meal, made up of everything you would ordinarily eat, but don't eat a mouthful of it. Instead, put it in a pot; then place the container with the food in a temperature around 100 degrees, the same as inside the body. See that there is a liberal quantity of moisture. Now watch what occurs over the next 8 hours.

The very first things you will notice are the bad odors and rancidity. Then the food will mold, ferment and bubble with gas. This gas pressure causes many miseries in the body. If the gas presses upward against the diaphragm you may even have stimulated a heart attack. As it presses against the back muscles, it can cause terrible backaches. This fermenting mass of putrefaction is always throwing off toxins which can cause pounding headaches, mysterious aches and pains all over the body.

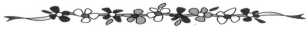

Dine with little, sup with less: do better still, sleep supperless. – Ben Franklin

Elementary microbiology tells us that, to produce germs in quantity, keep food fermenting in the colon and the bacteria will obligingly multiply. So, right in our bodies, we breed all kinds of "bugs" that can cause trouble. If you are prone to viruses such as colds, chronic sinusitis and other ailments, a constipated condition creates a favorable environment for the presence and growth of unfriendly "bugs" involved in such ailments.

The toxic poisons generated by overeating or too much of the wrong foods, can damage one of the body's most important organs – the liver. Few people realize how important their liver is to life. It's a great chemical laboratory with many functions. It not only gives forth bile, but it is the body's greatest garbage disposal.

The liver and intestines are partners in the whole digestive process! If one is sick, the other tries to come to its aid until it too, breaks down. When the liver and the digestive systems break down you are in serious trouble! This is why you often find a swollen sensitive liver, a pasty complexion and many times, jaundice and chronic fatigue in conjunction with ongoing constipation.

Give the Vital Force a Chance to Clean House!

So it's plain that when you stop eating to give your body's Vital Force a chance to clean house . . . you will miss the food habit the first few days of your fast! It could be uncomfortable if you allow it! Think positive!

When you fast, the Vital Force loosens the waste in your body and gathers it up to be discarded. As long as this goes on you might feel some discomfort. But once the waste is discarded through the kidneys, you will begin to feel better. As you fast, conditions change from day to day. When your body is eliminating heavy amounts of toxic poisons through the kidneys and other organs of elimination, you could feel some discomfort. But it should also be clear why you may feel better on the 7th day of a 10 day fast than you did on the 3rd day. Many of the toxic poisons that gave you trouble have been flushed out of the body! Many people who fast under my supervision felt far better and stronger on the 10th day of the fast than they did on the 1st day.

This always happens when I take a 7 or 10 day fast. I always feel stronger at the end of my fast than I did at the beginning. The cleaner you are inside, the more Vital Power you have! So at the beginning of the fast, just grin and bear the discomforts that may occur as you purify the body. You know that as you get cleaner, you are going to feel stronger. Whatever discomforts you may experience during a fast are well worth the great rewards you are going to receive! Again I say, to be a good faster, you must, "Just Grin and Bear It!"

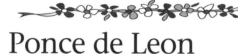

Ponce de Leon

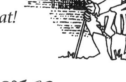

Searched for the
"Fountain of Youth."
If he had only known
It's within us . . .
Created by the food we eat!
Food can make or
Break your health!

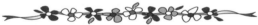

Perfection consists not in doing extraordinary things, but in doing ordinary things extraordinarily well. Neglect nothing; the most trivial action may be performed with joy. – Angelique Arnauld

---

The word "vegetarian" is not derived from "vegetable,"
but from the Latin, homo vegetus, meaning among the
Romans a strong, robust, thoroughly healthy man.

Liquefied and Fresh Juiced Foods

The juicer, food processor and blender are great for preparing foods for gentle (bland) diets and baby foods. Fibers of juiced fresh fruits and vegetables can be tolerated on most gentle diets. Any raw or cooked fruit or vegetable can be liquefied and added to broth, soups and non-dairy (soy, rice or nut) milks. Fresh juices supercharge your energy level and immune system to maximize your body's health power. You may fortify your liquid meal or Bragg Pep Drinks with any of these green powders for extra nutrition: alfalfa, chlorella, barley green, spirulina or wheat grass.

Chapter 13

Fasting Fights and Removes Mucus

In my opinion most of man's problems stem from a clogging of the entire pipe system of the human body. Most of this clogging takes the form of a thick mucus.

How free are you of mucus at this minute? Do you have a postnasal drip? That is, is there a slow dripping of mucus from your sinus cavities into the back of your mouth and down your throat? What about your nose? How much mucus are you carrying in your nasal passages? How many times a day do you use tissues? How many times a day do you clear your throat? How often do you cough or spit up mucus and phlegm?

Every person living on the average American diet has, more or less, a sticky mucus-clogged pipe system. This toxic mucus results from the undigested and uneliminated, unnatural food substances and toxins that start accumulating from birth. This mucus not only clogs the nose, throat and lungs, but this mucus is also found all along the 30 feet of the gastrointestinal tract that starts at the mouth and extends to the anus. Some humans suffer great distress from heavy mucus-clogging in their sinus cavities. It's found in the ears, not only in a soft form, but also in a hardened wax that can cause hearing problems. The greatest amount of mucus is most often lodged in the lungs.

Pneumonia is one of the most deadly diseases. Mucus fills up the lungs so you can't get enough air in to purify the 5 to 8 quarts of blood which flow to the lungs for vital purification. Pneumonia kills more older people; they literally drown in their own mucus.

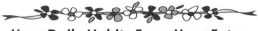

Your Daily Habits Form Your Future

Habits can be wrong, good or bad, healthy or unhealthy, rewarding or unrewarding. The right or wrong habits, decisions, actions, words or deeds . . . are up to you! Wisely choose your habits, as they can make or break your life! – Patricia Bragg

American Diet Forms Mucus and Illness

Our bodies are equipped with an elastic pipe system. The modern diet that we eat is never entirely digested and the accumulated waste never entirely eliminated. Our entire pipe system is slowly becoming clogged, especially the digestive tract. This is the foundation of many physical problems. The body becomes overloaded with mucus which the avenues of elimination cannot expel. It slowly concentrates into a huge decayed mass.

The American diet is a mucus-forming, heavily refined, high sugar, salt, fried foods, dairy, meats and fats diet. All dairy products are especially mucus-forming. No animal in the world except man drinks milk after being weaned. The modern diet includes butter and butter substitutes, margarines, processed shortenings and hydrogenated oils and fats which are the plugging saturated fats. These are unhealthy for the body. Our bodies have a normal temperature of 98.6°. To digest and assimilate these solid, hardened, saturated fats, we would have to have a heat of 300 degrees in our bodies. Our American diet contains a great deal of processed and synthetic cheese, as well as natural cheeses which are heavily preserved with salt. I have discussed the dangers of salt quite fully in this book. Don't use salt!

Most Americans love eggs, yet eggs carry large amounts of cholesterol, a saturated fat. If you eat eggs they should be fresh, fertile and from free range, organically fed chickens. Most Americans eat a lot of meat, most of it fried in heavy grease, either lard or hydrogenated commercial oils. Meat also carries its own heavy load of fat, both visible and invisible. In our modern civilization, much of our cooking is done by the deep-frying method, including Americans favorite food – french fries. You can see that this devitalized diet is a mucus-forming, unhealthy diet.

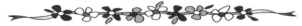

The greatest force in the human body is the natural drive of the body to heal itself – but that force is not independent of the belief system. Everything begins with belief. What we believe is the most powerful option of all. – Norman Cousins

Mucus Shows Up in the Urine when Fasting

The urine test shows the amount of mucus the average human carries within their bloodstream. Take a 3 day fast. Eat absolutely nothing and drink only large amounts of distilled water – from 2 to 3 quarts a day. Every morning of the fast, take a sample of the first urine you pass on awakening, put it in a labeled bottle and place it on a shelf to cool and settle. In a few days this urine will show a heavy cloud of mucus. The longer you keep the urine, the more toxins and mucus are revealed.

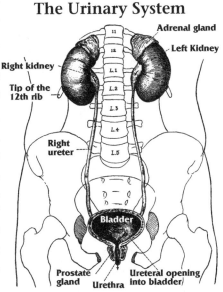

The Urinary System

Adrenal gland
Left Kidney
Right kidney
11
12
L1
L2
L3
L4
L5
Tip of the 12th rib
Right ureter
Bladder
Prostate gland
Urethra
Ureteral opening into bladder

A regular weekly 24 hour fast will help rid your body of large amounts of mucus and toxins. Some of these toxins have been circulating in your body for years.

In winter, most people eat more heavy, concentrated foods – such as refined flour products: pancakes, waffles, sugared cereals, doughnuts, rolls, breads, flour gravies, biscuits, cakes, pies and refined pastas – the body then becomes so loaded with mucus that it forces the Vital Force to create a cleansing crisis – a cold, flu, etc. A fever is produced by the Vital Force to help burn up and flush out the heavy concentrations of mucus. The lungs, nose and throat pour out the mucus through coughing, sneezing, spitting and nose-blowing. Few humans realize what a cleansing holocaust the body goes through!

The body is a miracle self-purifying instrument. As long as the body has enough Vital Force to eliminate toxins such as mucus, it will work with all its energy to rid and purify the body. What do humans think about this crisis? They get feverish. A fever is your body's cleaner, a true natural phenomenon of Mother Nature and acts as her incinerator to burn up the toxins.

Winter Miseries? Or Body Cleansing?

The uninformed man will tell you that he is suffering this winter misery because he got his feet wet! Or he will say that a draft blew on him and he didn't get his coat on in time. These are unscientific and weak excuses. Winter miseries, colds, flu, etc. are Mother Nature's internal self cleansing and purification blessings to help you get the mucus and toxins out and get healthy!

I have proven over and over that you can't catch colds. In the early years I was associated with Bernarr Macfadden, the father and founder of the Physical Culture Movement. He organized a group of people known as the Polar Bears. Every weekend and holiday in the frigid winter, we would meet at the Coney Island Beach in New York to frolic and exercise. Then we would all plunge into the icy water of the Atlantic Ocean.

Did I ever see one of the winter bathers ever have the sniffles? Never! People would come to Coney Island bundled up in heavy overcoats, mufflers, sweaters and flannel underwear to stand on the boardwalk, staring at us swimming and splashing around in the icy water. They were the people who had the sniffles, not the Polar Bears – who believed in eating a mucusless diet, exercising outdoors and swimming in icy waters.

Today I belong to two fine organizations who swim all year long at Coney Island, New York – the Polar Bears and the Icebergs. These two clubs are made up of men and women who are cold water swimmers. I also belong to the Winter Bathers Club (The Boston Brownies) who are headquartered at the "L" Street Bath House. Here is another group of people who prove that you can swim and expose yourself to the most frigid weather and still never have a sniffle, a chill, a fever or other reactions from exposure to cold weather. I live in California where the Pacific Ocean drops down to 50 degrees in winter. If I am not away on a lecture tour, you can count on me to take my cold water swims at the beach not far away.

Now I see the secret of the making of the best persons. It is to grow in the open air and eat and sleep with Mother Earth. – Walt Whitman

Take the Mucus Test

I feel that fasting has done a great deal to eliminate the mucus from my body. I faithfully live on a mucusless diet and always take my weekly 24 hour fast to help keep any mucus and toxins that I may have accumulated in my body flowing outward.

Take the test yourself! Eliminate all of the mucus-forming foods from your diet for several months. Fast 1 day a week and, if possible, take a 7 day fast. Watch your urine closely. See for yourself the amount of mucus you have concentrated in your body. After a fast, make 60% to 70% of your diet raw salads, vegetables and fruits and the balance in cooked vegetables, beans, legumes and brown rice. This is a mucusless diet that's rich in enzymes and nutrients. Also the raw, unsalted nuts and the nut butters and seeds (pumpkin, sunflower, sesame, etc.) are not mucus-forming, so add them to your diet of organic fruits and vegetables. While on this test don't eat any dairy, eggs, meats and only a few whole grains.

109

I can tell you all the great benefits that fasting, a mucusless and meatless diet will do for you. But it's best you simply try it yourself, then you be the judge. Notice how seldom you have to use a handkerchief. A 7 day fast is a great mucus eliminator. I make it a practice to fast a week to ten days in late October or November so that, as the winter comes on, I have relieved my body of any mucus that it has accumulated. I try to live on a mucusless diet. When traveling all over the world lecturing, I find that at times I can't get all the organic fruits and vegetables that I normally eat, so I put my faith in fasting for my internal purification.

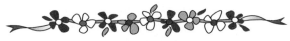

The treatment of diseases should go to the root cause, and most often it is found in severe dehydration from lack of sufficient pure, distilled water, plus an unhealthy lifestyle!

A good book goes around the world offering itself to reasonable men, who read it with joy and carry it to their reasonable neighbors. – Ralph Waldo Emerson

Breaking the Tobacco, Alcohol, Tea And Coffee Habit Through Fasting

It seems today most humans are addicted to some kind of poisonous drug habit – such as tobacco, alcohol, tea and coffee. Every one of these substances contain dangerous toxic poisons. The spotlight of science is still on the dangers of tobacco. Every cigarette package has this warning, "Tobacco smoking may be hazardous to your health." Scientists worldwide have studied the effects of tobacco on humans. The conclusion: smoking should be stopped! But it's not. Sad truth, *"Flesh is dumb and will accept anything."* Your mind must be a strong and faithful health captain to keep you healthy and fit!

The flesh will accept the carbon monoxide and nicotine of tobacco. It will accept alcohol. It will accept the caffeine tars found in coffee, tea and even chocolate. The body has no mechanism to process these vicious drugs and poisons. Millions are destroying their lives using these killers . . . it's like a slow, deliberate suicide.

Now, if a person wishes to release himself from the bondage of these irritating and poisonous drugs that act first to stimulate and then to depress the central nervous system, they must fast. The fast is a salvation for those who wish to break free of the shackles of these poisonous habits. In my years of supervising fasts, I have seen these wretched habits repeatedly defeated by fasting!

I remember years ago when a woman came to me who was a chain smoker. She smoked at least 4 packages of cigarettes a day and drank at least a fifth of whisky. She was a heavy user of coffee and colas. She told me her nerves were shattered. If she picked up a pencil to write, she trembled. She couldn't sleep. Her appetite was gone. Her eyes were blurred. Her skin tone was pasty and flabby. She was miserable and even had thoughts of suicide! Her physician suggested she see me, that I might help her with nutrition and exercise therapies to get some relief. She had reached the end of her rope and was willing to try anything. I love helping people who want to live and will follow The Bragg Healthy Lifestyle!

The Body Rebels Against Poisons!

The first thing I did with this smoking addict was to put her on a fast. I didn't take her poisons away from her. She continued to smoke and drink a small amount of alcohol and coffee. But on the third morning of her fast, her body rebelled and these stored poisons and toxins in her body began to nauseate her. The body wanted them out! When nauseated it's best to force it out by drinking 2-3 glasses of water, put your finger on the back of your tongue, lean over a bowl and get it out! You'll feel better right away! Every time she would light a cigarette or take any alcohol, tea or coffee she had heavy attacks of vomiting, nature's purge. I supervised the fast for 10 days. Those last 7 days of that fast were the first in years that she had not polluted her body with these deadly poisons. I broke her fast the tenth day and the urine she passed that morning was a thick ugly mass. Do you know what this mass was? – her poison residues. I then put her on a mucusless diet for 10 days and then fasted her again for 10 days. Every day of the second 10 day fast, large amounts of toxic poisons showed up in her urine.

I had her photographed at the start of her fast and at the end of 10 months. You would hardly know it was the same woman! Her skin and muscle tone were perfect. Her hands were firm and steady. Instead of a miserable, depressed human, she was now happy and carefree! She never again had the desire for tobacco, alcohol, tea or coffee. She became one of the best writers in the Hollywood TV and movie world. Her income doubled and tripled. Her personal magnetism increased and she attracted a handsome, wholesome man for a husband.

The list is long of people who had hit rock bottom with their addictions who then turned to fasting as a last resort – and fasting did the trick! Any person who is addicted to tobacco, alcohol, drugs, tea or coffee, etc. will find an answer to their problems by fasting. When the body becomes clean, it will no longer allow poisons to enter. A pure, clean, wholesome body and strong mind will always reject poisons. Fasting is the greatest method to purify the body and to keep it healthy and strong!

⟨ DEADLY SMOKING FACTS! ⟩

✞ Tobacco use and secondhand smoke will eventually kill just over ⅕ of all the people now living in the developed world – over 250 million.

✞ Of the 50 million smoking Americans, ⅓ to ½ will die from smoke-related disease, and reduce their life expectancy by an average of 9 years.

✞ Cancers, as well as cataracts, are linked to smoking.

✞ Children and teenagers make up 90% of new smokers in the US – and teenage smoking is on the rise.

✞ Smoking acts as both a stimulant and a depressant - depending upon the smoker's emotional state.

✞ The average pack-a-day smoker takes about 70,000 *poisonous hits* of nicotine each year.

✞ "Secondhand smoke" can kill nonsmokers: it speeds up heart rate, raises blood pressure and doubles the carbon monoxide in their blood.

✞ Secondary smoke contains more nicotine, tar and cadmium (leading to hypertension, bronchitis and emphysema) than mainstream smoke.

✞ The children of smokers tend to have lower body weight and smaller lungs.

✞ Lung illnesses such as asthma are twice as common in the children of smokers.

✞ The death rate from breast cancer ranges from 25% to 75% higher for women who smoke.

✞ Female smokers may face a higher risk of lung cancer – as much as twice the risk of male smokers, according to a study done by Dr. Harvey Risch at Yale University.

✞ Your body contains almost 100,000 miles of blood vessels. Smoking constricts those vessels, depriving your body of the fresh, rich oxygen it needs.

> **QUIT SMOKING!** In just 12 hours of not smoking, blood levels of nicotine and carbon monoxide fall; heart and lungs begin healing. Smokers must stop this vicious and deadly destroyer of life, health, energy and beauty.

Chapter 14

Fasting Melts Away Pounds!

It's estimated that 75% of men, women and children in America are overweight. These overweight people are in serious physical trouble according to medical authorities and insurance companies. Excess weight presents great hazards to health and long life. These same authorities tell us that the overweight person is more susceptible to chronic and even fatal diseases than a normal weight person. An overweight person can't begin to know the thrill of wellness. First, they are constantly tired because they are carrying far too many pounds. Let's say a person is 25 pounds overweight. Now, let a normal weight person carry a 25 pound suitcase around all day. In a short time every move would become painful and fatiguing. You can plainly see overweight people have overburdened their bodies.

113

The obese person typically has no ambition to indulge in physical activities. Most of them would rather find the closest chair and sit in it until they are forced to do some important duty. The overweight person has trouble breathing because their excess flesh makes it difficult for their lungs to do their jobs properly, so we find them out of breath at the least exertion.

The overweight person's body has over 700 miles (unbelievable, but true) of fine tubes – blood vessels – to try and nourish and sustain all the excess fat! You can plainly see why the overweight person is putting a tremendous burden on the lungs and the normal function of their heart. Their pulse and blood pressure rise to dangerous heights, which could in themselves cause serious damage, heart attacks, strokes and death.

Every man is the builder of a temple called his body . . . We are all sculptors and painters, and our material is our own flesh and blood and bones. Any nobleness begins at once to refine a man's features, any meanness to imbrute them. – Henry David Thoreau

Fat is a Burden and Health Risk!

Insurance figures accurately show that overweight people are short-lived and are more susceptible to many chronic diseases because of their unnatural overweight condition. Any way you look at it, excess weight is dangerous! Today, obesity is steadily on the increase worldwide. First, in America we have an abundance of food and fast food restaurants. The average person puts way too much food into their stomach for the sheer joy of eating. Eating is America's most popular indoor and outdoor sport! Family gatherings call for many varieties of food. When people entertain their relatives and friends there is always a tendency to serve too much variety and everyone overeats.

Coffee breaks encourage people to snack between meals. TV invites people to snack as they gaze at the idiot box that promotes crime and evilness. Plus people are constantly eating sweets, ice cream, shakes, hot dogs, hamburgers, french fries, pizza and many other varieties of food even between meals. Then there are the buffets, banquets, benefit dinners, etc. that promote overeating.

We live in a mechanical age. We load heavy amounts of food into our bodies and never burn it up with exercise and physical activities. The automobile has replaced walking. We are a nation of sitters. Our children sit for hours in school and then in front of the TV. People spend hours at computers, attending movies, concerts, athletic events and musicals. This unhealthy, sedentary life contributes to being overweight.

Fad Diets Create Up and Down Weight

Overweight people are constantly going on crash diets and most get only brief results. There is the high-protein diet, the low-carbohydrate diet, the liquid diet, the cottage cheese diet, etc., etc. and so many other varieties. Magazines and newspapers are always pushing some new crash diet to take weight off the obese person.

There are so many reducing diets that it's frustrating and confusing for people to know which one to follow. In my opinion, the fast is the only natural and scientific way to achieve reasonable weight reduction. Let me give you some of my reasons why I believe fasting is the perfect way to reduce. After the first 2 or 3 days of fasting you are no longer hungry. From the 3rd day on there is no craving for food. When people go on crash diets that are low calorie, they are hungry most of the time and long for heavy meals. But after you fast for 2 or 3 days, all hunger fades away, the stomach shrinks and it actually becomes a very pleasant experience. You start to breathe easier, feel lighter, move easier and think more clearly.

Fasting Rewards You With Increased Energy

I have seen many overweight people lose 7 to 20 pounds and more the first 7 to 10 days of fasting. After the loss of this excess weight, there is a special inner feeling of well-being and increased physical and mental energy! Of course, every human is different. Some people only lose 1 or 2 pounds a day on a fast while some will lose as many as 5 pounds.

The nice thing about fasting to reduce is that the pounds disappear where the fat is deposited. If the weight has concentrated on the abdomen and hips, that is where the fat will shrink. Many times the people who go on a low calorie diet end up feeling miserable while they are dieting. They become haggard and old-looking and their eyes will lose their sparkle. It is just the reverse when you fast. The fat deposits dissolve first and – as the body is relieved of this tremendous burden – the heart, pulse and blood pressure will regulate themselves.

So, if you have a weight problem, use this Fasting Program. You can start with a weekly 24 hour fast. I often supervise weight reduction programs, where I direct people on several 36 hour fasts in a week. In other words, they will eat 1 day, then fast a day or fast every third day. If the person doesn't overload himself on the days he eats, the 36 hour fast several times a week helps him maintain the weight loss. Fasting for weight reduction does get results. Your body slims and trims itself back to its healthy, youthful lines again.

Good health and good sense are two of life's greatest blessings. – P. Syrus

Your Waistline is Your Lifeline & Dateline!

I have had years of experience in fasting many of our greatest film and television Stars in Hollywood, California. The movie camera always makes a person look 10 pounds heavier than they really are, so you can see that a Star must always have slim, trim lines!

I recall a well-known female movie Star who became a compulsive eater because she was having marital and financial troubles. She sought solace in eating rich foods such as ice cream, heavily sugared pastries and candies. In time she lost her movie contract because of her overweight. She was a good actress, but the public makes severe demands on their heroes! This actress became depressed and had to seek the services of a psychiatrist. The psychiatrist then sent this actress to me for guidance. I explained to this actress it had taken months for her to add this weight to her body and it would now take time to slim, trim and normalize her weight. She was determined to lose weight, so she was most cooperative!

First, I put her on a good diet program with fruit for breakfast, a raw salad with 2 lightly cooked vegetables – such as string beans, carrots, squash, collards or stewed tomatoes – for lunch. I took all bread, cereals and animal proteins out of her diet. In the evening she had the Bragg Health Salad and the brown rice and lentil casserole (recipes page 231). Naturally, sugar desserts were eliminated.

I started her on 2 weekly 24 hour fasts for the first 2 weeks. The third week I gave her a 3 day fast and in the fifth week I gave her a full 7 day fast. After a month of healthy eating I put her on a 15 day fast. I had her eat for 2 weeks and then put her on a 21 day fast. This eating, then fasting program did the trick! She got back her lovely figure. (5'2" and a trim 110 pounds.) Her eyes became bright and clear and she regained her youthful appearance. Producers, directors, friends were amazed.

Fasting provides the magic formula for retaining youthful beauty and a streamlined body!

Even if I knew certainly the world would end tomorrow, I would plant an apple tree today. – Martin Luther

Fasting – A Challenge To
Improve Your Health and Looks

Yes, it's a challenge because our eating habits are so ingrained in our consciousness that fasting to many humans is akin to starvation. It is not starvation. Fasting is one of the oldest remedies known to man. So I say again, the mind must control the flesh! "Flesh is dumb!"

It takes intelligence, logic and reasoning to know when to turn down food. If you are a determined person, if you believe in the law of compensation, you will make fasting an important part of your life. Don't let excess weight make you a sick, old, unhealthy, unattractive person! Revolt against fat. Be the captain of your body! Say to yourself, "I am no longer going to be burdened with unhealthy, sick, flabby flesh!" Work out an exercise and fasting program for yourself, and don't try to get the fat off in a week. It took a long time to get heavy and it will take a reasonable length of time to melt it away. You will be so proud of yourself when you slim and trim yourself down to your normal weight with normal measurements. Your family and friends will also.

117

Every person is aware of their health and physical appearance! We all want to look and feel our best. So let's do something about it! Fasting and sensible, sane dieting and exercise is your answer! Be sure you have a bathroom scale and get yourself a tape measure. Weigh yourself and measure your abdomen, hips, thighs and arms. With determination commit yourself to a serious program of normalizing your weight for health's sake!

To prove the value of fasting to yourself, get a physical exam before starting your fasting regimen and get copies of your blood/cholesterol panel test (see page 138), urine etc. for your home medical files. After faithfully following The Bragg Healthy Lifestyle with fasting you will be amazed at the improvements you have gained.

Fasting is always the best way to take off fat; I am not going to tell you fasting is always easy. It's going to take positive thinking and action to attain positive results! Start today to lose any dangerous excess pounds!

Do these Exercises Daily (10 per set):

You must exercise, for weak muscles of the arms, legs and entire body indicates a similar condition of the stomach and heart (a muscle) and other organs.

> **Important Exercises for Keeping the External and Internal Muscles of The Stomach Fit and Healthy. Also These Promote Good Elimination.**

Bend at the waist to the sides, then front and back.

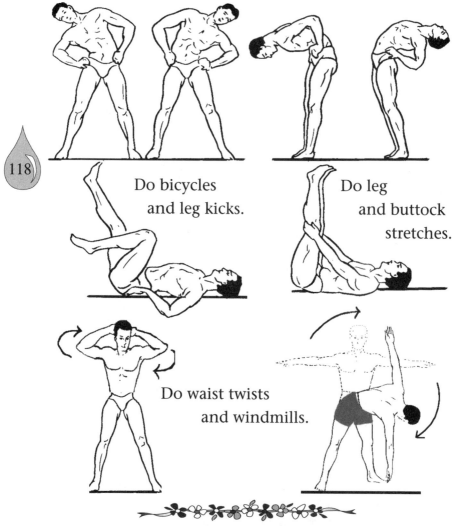

Do bicycles and leg kicks.

Do leg and buttock stretches.

Do waist twists and windmills.

Exercise, along with fasting, is provided to help us maintain or restore a healthy physical balance in our daily living for a long, happy life.

Chapter 15

How to Gain Weight Using a Scientific Fasting Program

Thin people fight frantically to gain and hold a few pounds. Gaining weight becomes an obsession with the underweight person and they are most susceptible to all kinds of weight-gaining diets. Underweight people have come to me in a frustrated and emotional condition, begging me to help them put a few pounds on their spare frames. Most of them were cold constantly . . . even on the warmest summer days they wore sweaters and heavy garments! They begged me to give them a diet that would help them gain weight, because they were ashamed of their skeleton-like bodies.

When I told them there was no such thing as a weight-gaining diet, they were as shocked as if I had given them a death sentence. But, when I added most emphatically that there was a program to gain weight which included fasting, they would agree to the program but not on the fasting! They would cry out, "Don't make me any thinner than I am! I'm down to skin and bones now. If you take my food away from me, I will look like a scarecrow!" Then I had to explain that they were thin only because their bodies were nutritionally unbalanced.

I told them that food and nutrition are not synonymous. A diet of unhealthy fats, refined sugar, and carbohydrates, plus ample milk, cream and more fattening foods wouldn't necessarily help them gain weight; their body might even get thinner on this diet. They must cleanse and heal their body by fasting and living a healthy lifestyle and take a multi-enzyme.

Famous comedian & author Dick Gregory, who weighed 320 pounds, was inspired by our Miracle of Fasting *book that guided him into a healthy lifestyle which was life-changing. He traded his bad habits – unhealthy foods, alcohol, drugs, smoking, etc. for healthy habits!!! He now weighs a healthy 150 pounds and has been in 8 Boston Marathons and is guiding others to reduce and live on "live foods" and abstain from unhealthy, processed foods.*

People are not nourished in proportion to the amount of food they eat, but in proportion to how much they digest and assimilate. When the organs of digestion and assimilation are maintained in poor working condition, eating too many fatty foods in an effort to gain weight defeats its own purpose.

Being underweight is usually due to faulty health. It's futile to stuff a lot of food into the body when assimilation and digestion are working at a low ebb. The secret of normalizing weight (up or down) is to make the detoxifying system more efficient through fasting. Then the underweight person rejuvenates the digestive and assimilative systems to work efficiently.

What the underweight person needs is exactly what the overweight person needs – a fast that gives the body a physiological rest. In both the overweight and the underweight, the digestive and assimilation systems have been overworked. This is difficult to explain to underweight people. They are impatient and want to gain weight immediately on a diet, but first the underweight person must realize that the period of physiological rest provided by the fast results in improved digestion and assimilation of foods.

The Body Has Recuperative Powers

The body has extraordinary recuperative powers when it is not burdened with an excessive amount of food. In over 70 years of fasting underweight people, I have had outstanding success with underweight and emaciated people who learned to have faith in fasting and a full program of Natural Living.

I have a sister whom I love very dearly who was born a very tiny baby. I believe she weighed about 3 pounds at birth. All through her life, my sister Louise was called "skinny." When she was a child, everyone would tell my mother that she should be stuffed with milk and cream and that she must eat a lot of pork, potatoes, rice, custards and all the supposed weight-gaining foods. But the more my sister was stuffed with all of these so-called fattening foods, the thinner, weaker, paler and more lifeless she became! There were many times when my sister was so weak that she had to remain in bed. And even during these periods in bed, she was still stuffed on a so-called weight-gaining diet.

Later, after I had left home and regained my health, I returned to Virginia near where my sister Louise lived. She was then an adult and unmarried. She was teaching high school and was thin, rundown and had an overall weakness. Her color was ghastly. After a hard day in the classroom, she would come home and throw herself across the bed in a state of exhaustion.

I told her that I had found a natural way for people to gain weight and when school closed and summer vacation began, I would return to Virginia and supervise a program to help her gain weight. She had seen the great miracle that had transformed my body after I began living the natural life and had perfect confidence in everything I told her. I explained to her that part of the program would be a series of fasts which would give her body a physiological rest. This would allow the digestive and the assimilative organs of her body a chance to revive and rejuvenate themselves.

This is a cleansing system of detoxification. I told her that the fast would help increase the hydrochloric acid in her stomach so that she could absorb more protein foods. Not only would the digestion of protein be better, but all the digestive organs would improve and renew themselves through the fast. Her whole process of metabolism would improve through her fasting program.

I have proved over the years that when metabolism is improved through fasting there is a healthier density and a specific gravity in the new flesh that is built after fasting. The fast assists the body to assimilate proteins, fats, carbohydrates, starches, sugars, minerals, vitamins and all the other essential nutrients necessary for the body to work efficiently and with more strength.

Good! You have decided to take the Health and Happiness road to Higher Health. There will be a few rough spots as you begin, but soon you will be hiking along the Pathway of Health and Long-Lasting Youthfulness!

Miracles Happen With Fasting!

I started Louise on a 7 day distilled water fast. She entered this fast believing that Mother Nature was going to purify her digestive and assimilative organs and help her rebuild a new body. It is true that she lost weight in the 7 days of the fast, but after she broke the fast she developed a healthy appetite. What miracles this week of rest for her organs did for her system. She told me she had never enjoyed food as much as she now was enjoying her new diet. Not the so-called "good, nourishing, fattening food," but a diet of 60% raw, fresh salads, vegetables and luscious, fresh fruits and brown rice, lentils and raw nuts and seeds, etc. I gave her cooked vegetables and beans, brown rice and lentils, raw, unsalted nuts and seeds and their butters. A month after the first fast, I put her on another fast of 7 days. This 7 day fast started a new life for her because her body was in such clean, healthy condition that it began to fill out.

My skinny sister became a beautiful woman – fully rounded and streamlined – every part of her body seemed to be rejuvenated. Her hair took on a sheen it never had before, there was a glow to her cheeks and a sparkle in her eyes like a young child! Our relatives and friends were flabbergasted at the transformation in Louise. The happiest part is that within a year my sister had become one of the most popular girls in Westmoreland County, Virginia, and in another year she had married a fine, handsome man! Their lives were like a fairy tale because they had children and lived happily ever after. My sister also remained healthy, fit and youthful.

Along with fasting, I gave my sister a system of exercises. She started with short walks and then built up to long walks. I persuaded her to get an abundance of fresh air, take early morning or late afternoon sunbaths and do deep breathing exercises. At all times, she maintained a tranquil and serene mind . . . she worked with Mother Nature and not against her!

Eat not for the pleasure thou mayest find therein; eat to increase thy strength, eat to preserve the life thou hast received from Heaven.
– Confucius

Fasting is a Weight Normalizer

What I did for my weak, thin sister, I have done for thousands of underweight people. Fasting works miracles for both the under and overweight. The genuine needs for both types of people are met by exactly the same program of natural living combined with fasting.

Fasting is the magic key for helping anyone to restore themselves to a superior state of health. Fasting is the great detoxifier and by detoxifying the body we give it a chance to restore its normal functioning. Fasting is the great "Open Sesame" to good health and long life.

Each person is different and some get results quicker than others. If you really concentrate on living The Bragg Healthy Lifestyle in which fasting plays an integral part, Mother Nature will never fail you! So, if you are thin and underweight and have tried all sorts of weight-building diets that failed, don't be discouraged. Instead, try a program of fasting. Give Mother Nature a chance to make you a person of normal weight.

123

The doctor of the future will give no medicine but will interest his patients in the care of the human frame, in diet, and in the cause and prevention of disease

Thomas A. Edison

Morning Resolve

I will this day live a simple, sincere and serene life, repelling promptly every thought of impurity, discontent, anxiety, discouragement and self-seeking. I will cultivate cheerfulness, happiness, charity and the love of brotherhood; exercising economy in expenditure, generosity in giving, carefulness in conversation and diligence in appointed service. I pledge fidelity to every trust and a childlike faith in God. In particular, I will be faithful in those habits of prayer, study, work, physical exercise, deep breathing and good posture. I shall fast one 24 hour period each week, eat only natural foods and get sufficient sleep each night. I will make every effort to improve myself physically, mentally, emotionally and spiritually every day.

Morning Prayer used by Paul C. Bragg and Patricia Bragg

Dr. Oliver Wendell Holmes declared that if all the doctor's drugs were thrown into the sea it would be so much better for humankind and worse for the fish.

Cheerfulness and content are great beautifiers and are famous preservers of youthful looks. – Charles Dickens

Everyday is a birthday; every moment of it is new to us; we are born again, renewed for fresh work and endeavor. – Isaac Watts

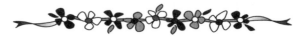

Give us Lord, a bit of sun,
A bit of work and a bit of fun.
Give us, in all struggle and sputter,
Our daily whole grain bread and food.
Give us health, our keep to make
And a bit to spare for others' sake.
Give us too, a bit of song
And a tale and a book, to help us along.
Give us Lord, a chance to be
Our goodly best for ourselves and others
Until men learn to live as brothers.

– An Old English Prayer

Chapter 16

Fasting Fights Winter Miseries

No matter how well and healthy you try to live, colds, sniffles and flu will catch up with you. If this happens, please don't be discouraged, but be thankful your body is house cleaning.

When your nose drips hot, watery mucus and your head feels thick while you sneeze; when fever burns through your body and you feel terrible, don't blame it on the weather! Don't blame it on a cold draft of air! Don't blame it on the fact that you got your feet wet or that you got chilled! And above all things, don't say, "I caught it!" The proper name for this is an "acute healing crisis." The reason we go through this is that we live in a complex civilization and we have lost so much of our natural instinct to keep internally pure.

So – for some physiological reason that is absolutely unexplainable – the Vital Force within our bodies loosens up waste, toxins and mucus and proceeds to get rid of it with the "acute healing crisis (colds, flu, etc.)." If you cooperate with your Vital Force, this rough spot in your life will pass away quickly. So don't blame it on a vicious little bug, a virus or cold weather. Just understand that your Vital Force is trying to keep you internally clean.

If you interfere with Mother Nature, you will complicate the whole procedure of your body's miraculous cleansing job. Now that you know why this acute healing crisis occurs, you should do nothing to stop the cleansing process except to fast. Yes, that's the simple and best answer – fast and help cleanse your body!

You must not fight this healing crisis because Mother Nature knows what she is doing for you. What should you do? Start your fasting program right away! There is absolutely nothing as important as your health and life!

A prayer in its simplest definition is merely a wish turned God-ward.
– Phillips Brooks

Fast and Rest For Your Healing!

Drop everything you are doing and get into a warm bed. Stop all eating. That also means no fruit or fruit juices. At regular intervals drink large amounts of hot, distilled water with just a little honey with lemon juice or apple cider vinegar. Eat and drink nothing else. See that you have a good circulation of pure air in your bedroom. Don't read, listen to the radio or watch TV! Just sleep and rest – nothing else. Above all, don't waste precious energy talking to relatives and friends! Go into complete seclusion to cleanse and recharge. You are on God's cleansing table.

How long should you fast during a winter healing crisis or, for that matter, a summer healing crisis? They can happen at any time of the year, but generally strike in cold weather. In most instances, 3 days of restful fasting will put you on your feet again. But sometimes it may take a week or 10 days to do a successful job. Don't quibble about it! You will find that you will be in better health after the healing crisis. If you will work with your Vital Force, you will flush out a tremendous amount of internal poison. Just don't panic! Mother Nature is very wise and she knows what is best for you.

If you have faith and confidence in Mother Nature, you will always work with her. I reared 5 children and when the sniffles hit them, I had them fast and rest. In a few days they would snap out of the healing crisis and be their same robust selves again. My grandchildren followed this program . . . and now my great-grandchildren are following it! To most people this program seems too simple – they feel that they must do or take something. They are filled with fear.

There is absolutely nothing to fear as long as Mother Nature is working to keep you alive and healthy. She knows best and will see you through any crisis, because she is God's own physician!

Each person should regard his health as the most precious blessing that he can possess and should attempt to understand his body which is so "fearfully and wonderfully made." He should maintain his precious body in Supreme Health as 3 John 2 states.

The Body is Self-Healing & Self-Repairing

Every man is not only the "Master Builder" of his character, but also the custodian of his health and physical well-being. Not only has the Creator endowed man with a "God-like" body, but He has given him a wonderful mind and reasoning power. Humans are capable of comprehending and putting to use all the natural resources for self-health and self-healing which have been so generously placed at their disposal.

The Miracle of Fasting is another way to help yourself to Higher Health. Mother Nature gives us simple healing remedies. We must be willing to cooperate with Mother Nature and conform our lives to her unchangeable laws. Following the "Natural Way of Living" we can recapture the precious bloom of youth through the gifts of physical, mental and spiritual regeneration. There are no shortcuts to health! Mother Nature expects us to do our part. When you fast you are working with Mother Nature. God and Mother Nature won't perform a miracle until we are willing to bring our lives and habits into conformity with Their Eternal Laws of Health.

It's my honest and sincere belief that nobody should ever promise to cure anyone of their physical misery. To promise anyone a cure means that someone is trying to play both God and Mother Nature and no human can promise you the results that They can perform!

By combining fasting with eating only healthy, natural foods, you can attain a more youthful, healthful life. Healing is an internal biological function that only the body can perform. By fasting you are helping your body do its cleansing work efficiently. Mother Nature is continually working to keep you alive and well. So when Mother Nature starts a healing crisis (colds, flu, etc.) she knows what she is doing. So be thankful and fast.

Fasting is the greatest assistance you can provide your body, because you are letting all of your Vital Force push the toxic poisons out of your entire body so you can be cleaner and healthier and more youthful!

Fasting is for internal cleansing, purification, staying healthy and youthful.

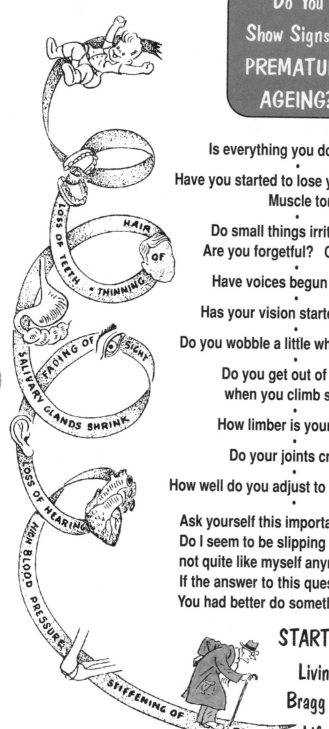

Is everything you do a big effort?

•

Have you started to lose your skin tone?
Muscle tone?

•

Do small things irritate you?
Are you forgetful?   Confused?

•

Have voices begun to fade?

•

Has your vision started to dim?

•

Do you wobble a little when you walk?

•

Do you get out of breath
when you climb stairs?

•

How limber is your back?

•

Do your joints creak?

•

How well do you adjust to cold and heat?

•

Ask yourself this important question:
Do I seem to be slipping and
not quite like myself anymore?
If the answer to this question is "Yes,"
You had better do something about it!

START TODAY
Living The
Bragg Healthy
Lifestyle!

He who understands nature walks with God. – Edgar Cayce

Chapter 17

Outwit Premature Ageing

Take This Quiz and The Mirror Test Now & Each Month After to Monitor Your Well-Being

Go to your mirror nude now and take the Mirror Test. Are you happy with what you see? • Do you look old and tired? • Does your body sag? • Do you have poor skin and muscle tone? • How's your hair? • How's your posture? • Are your eyes dull and lifeless? • Do you have a pale, sallow complexion? • Are you trim and fit?

After making a careful examination of your body, how would you describe it? • Youthful? • Ageing? No one can answer these questions more honestly than you. You're the only one that can take charge of your life!

Let us go farther than mere looks. How do you really feel today? • Are you bursting with energy and vitality or do you have bothersome aches and pains? • What about the moveable joints of your body? • Are you stiff and sore? • Does your lower back plague you with pain? • How did you sleep last night? • Did you get up fresh and feeling alive? • Did you go to bed tired, yet unable to sleep? • Did you face the new day feeling energyless as if all your energy had drained away? • How is your appetite? • Do you relish every mouthful of food you eat? • Are you plagued with gas pains after meals? • What about your elimination? • Is it perfect or are your bowels clogged? • Above all things, were you happy today? • Yesterday? • Or are you depressed and blue?

• Do you feel that you are ageing rapidly? • Is life passing you by? • Can you honestly say, "I am getting younger as I live longer?" • Or will you have to admit that the longer you live, the older you feel? • I know you want to look and feel youthful and not get old before your time. • So begin NOW to live The Bragg Healthy Lifestyle! You will see results – take this quiz monthly.

129

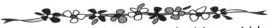

Nature, time and patience are three great physicians. – Irish Proverb

Fasting is a Miraculous Rebirth!

Let me tell you honestly what fasting can do for you. This natural miracle can help reverse the premature ageing process for you. From this minute on, you could take a new lease on life! It has been proven by some of the world's greatest scientists that fasting is the magic key that opens the door to agelessness and youthfulness.

Scientists have been experimenting for years on worms, white rats and guinea pigs, and they have discovered some remarkable scientific facts. They fasted these laboratory animals and, in between fasts, they fed them scientifically balanced, natural diets. A miracle occurred that almost sounds like a fairy tale . . . they got younger! These scientists are single-minded and want only facts, and the facts revealed the truth. All these findings have been published and you need only go to a good library to find these miraculous, vital discoveries!

Fasting not only slows down the ageing clock, but it produces a healthy youthfulness and rebirth in the body. In my years supervising fasts, I have seen thousands of almost unbelievable miracles happen to people all ages.

I remember a Bragg health student named Martin Cornica who had spent many years working in the film industry. He was about 40 when he realized he was ageing prematurely. He regarded himself as a middle-aged man. And why shouldn't he? Since the average life expectancy of an American male today is 78 years of age, he decided that at 40 he had lived over half his life. So he slowed his pace to that of a typical middle-aged man.

In his younger days Martin Cornica had been a champion tennis player. But he had discarded his tennis racket because he felt the game was only for the very young. Then someone at 20th Century Studio told him about The Bragg Health Crusade. Martin said that out of sheer curiosity, he attended one and it was the turning point in his life. It was the lifesaver that introduced him to continual youthfulness and endless energy.

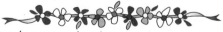

A book is a garden, an orchard, a storehouse, a party, a mentor, a teacher, a guidepost and a counsellor. – Henry Ward Beecher

Recharged, So at 70 World Tennis Champ

Martin Cornica learned the same facts that I have given to thousands of people all over the world. When you know the science of taking care of the body, you have the secret of a naturally healthy and youthful life. Martin wanted to look and feel youthful. He was eager to try Mother Nature's plan of living as I taught it.

He went on a 24 hour fast the day after he attended my Health Lecture. He began to eat a natural, wholesome and perfectly balanced diet. Through fasting and natural living he dropped years from his age. Even though he was 40 years old and considered long past the age to play strenuous tennis, Mr. Cornica felt stronger than when he was 20! His energy and vitality was super, so he joined the Los Angeles Tennis Club and started to play again. He continued to do this weekly 24 hour fast and live on a natural food diet. Every day he improved in every way. His endurance soon was so great that he was playing the champion tennis players of the world! For the next 30 years he played in one major tournament after another and won many championships. Tennis is often seen as a game for only the young and vigorous, but here was a man supposedly long past his prime playing with young champions and winning!

Martin Cornica became The Champion Tennis Player of the World for all men over 70! People in the tennis world were completely amazed when they saw this man in his 70s playing a smashing, championship tennis game.

The average person believes that by the time a man is 70 he is either half dead or used up. Martin Cornica is the living proof that this is a fallacy! It's not the number of years you live on this earth, it is how you have lived! I am very proud because he has absolutely proven that anyone can attain agelessness and be reborn by following Mother Nature's and God's Laws of Living. Regardless of your age, Mother Nature will give you the opportunity to make a comeback. Yes, you can step out of that tired, prematurely ageing body and rebuild a strong body that will become healthier and more youthful!

No one can violate Nature's Laws & escape her penalties. – Julian Johnson

After a year of periodic fasting combined with living The Bragg Healthy Lifestyle, you can look in the mirror and be happy with the big improvement you have made. If you continue to live The Bragg Healthy Lifestyle as described in this book, the physical transformation will make your friends and relatives take notice and marvel at your wonderful rejuvenation. You will not only see the difference in yourself, you will feel the difference! But you can only make this metamorphosis if you are willing to exercise absolute mastery of your body.

Start as Martin Cornica did with a 24 hour fast. Read the chapter on correct eating. The 9 Doctors of Mother Nature will aid you in your rebirth. They are always ready and willing to help those who help themselves.

There is just one sad note that I must mention. As you get younger and more vital, you will see those you love the most begin to decay and pass out of this life long before their time because they refused to learn the "greatest law of life," which is "The Survival of the Fittest." The same thing has happened in my personal life. I have had to watch the people I loved the most sicken, suffer and die long before their time simply because they would not live a healthy lifestyle.

The Opportunity of Your Lifetime

Revolt! Refuse to grow old! Refuse to lose precious years of your life! Mother Nature is waiting for you to make your decision this minute!

Good! You have decided to take the Health and Happiness road to Higher Health. There will be a few rough spots as you begin, but soon you'll be hiking along the Highway of Health and Long Lasting Youthfulness!

You cannot fail! You are working with God and Mother Nature and these are forces that will never, ever fail you. Begin your 24 hour fast today. You will soon laugh at birthdays. They will mean nothing to you! You are beginning to live in the blessed state of Agelessness!

Let food be your medicine, and medicine be your food. – Hippocrates

Chapter 18

Fasting Keeps the Arteries Young

Cardiovascular disease is responsible for 42% of the deaths in the United States, according to the American Heart Association. This should alarm you! Often we are shocked to hear that 200 people have died in an airplane crash, but are blasé about the fact that each day 2,600 Americans die from this disease! Disease of the heart, arteries and blood vessels is not only epidemic in America, it's the #1 killer! This enemy of mankind targets men and women, the old and the young! More than 1 in 4 Americans is currently suffering from some sort of cardiovascular disease! During the Korean, Vietnam and Gulf Wars, autopsies revealed that many young service people suffered from deteriorated and degenerated arteries – sadly, long before their time!

Diseases of the heart do not build up rapidly. It takes a long time to harden and block an artery! Heart disease has many causes . . . tobacco, alcohol, an unhealthy diet heavy in hydrogenated and saturated fats such as those in meats and dairy products and lack of exercise. Heart disease is a silent killer! Too frequently, blockage in the arteries is built up to the danger point while the victim is totally unaware! It is possible for a person to have half-blocked arteries all over their body without the slightest indication that anything is wrong. This person might even receive a clean bill of health from the best doctors! This happened to one of our past American Presidents – 1 week after a thorough physical with a good health report, he had a major heart attack!

The substances responsible for obstructing the arteries are cholesterol, fats, inorganic minerals and fibrous tissues. As the blockage builds up slowly, the inner passages of the arteries can become so narrow that not enough blood can flow through to properly nourish the powerful heart muscle. Coronary occlusion is caused when this serious narrowing of the arteries occurs.

You Are as Old as Your Arteries

Degeneration of the arteries begins early in life, slowly building up to obstruct and block! Then, one fine morning, someone gets up as usual to start the day's activities and suddenly, in the blink of an eye, they drop dead from a heart attack or must live with a very serious chronic condition after the attack.

Constant vigilance must be maintained if the arteries are to be kept free of blockage and obstruction by substances that can cause a heart attack. The heart arteries are small; the largest is no wider than a thin soda straw. In the average person who eats the average diet of today, the blockage grows silently, insidiously until the blood can no longer flow freely through the great arteries and disaster strikes.

Most people wait until something happens to their arteries before they do anything about it. Because no pains are evident, they continue to eat the bad food and live with the bad habits that destroy their arteries.

Again let me repeat the statement, "We are all as old as our arteries." Remember that arterial blockage starts even in the very young and slowly builds up until around 55 years of age, when most heart disasters take place.

I want it definitely understood that I do not believe that fasting is a cure for heart trouble. Fasting is a preventive health measure because, as I have continually stated in this book, fasting is a cleanser of internal impurities. This is exactly how we want to help our arteries – to keep them clean and free of substances that prevent the free flow of blood into the heart and throughout the entire arterial system.

Shocking Heart Facts About the #1 Killer

- *Cardiovascular diseases claimed over a million lives in the United States last year, accounting for almost half of all deaths!*

- *Every 33 seconds another American dies from cardiovascular disease!*

- *Heart disease doesn't just kill the old; 1 out of every 6 is under 65!*

- *Heart disease affects both men and women; lately men accounted for 49% of heart related fatalities, while women accounted for 51%.*

Don't let cardiovascular disease affect you! Protect your heart!

What You Eat and Drink Becomes You

We have, in the final analysis, a human pipe system that carries our precious 5 quarts of blood throughout the entire circulatory system. Our blood circulation must be kept constantly moving, rhythmically and steadily. For instance, if the flow of blood into the brain is stopped for a fraction of a minute, we could suffer a massive stroke. If it happens in the eye, hemorrhaging can occur that may blind us. The arteries must remain open so the bloodstream will flow to every square inch of the body.

Today you will find men and women in their 70s, 80s and even 90s who have clear, clean, unobstructed, elastic and flexible arteries. Regardless of their calendar years, they are young because their arteries have not degenerated to the point of becoming obstructed and inflexible. These are the most fortunate people in the world because if all the organs of their bodies are free from obstruction and toxic materials, there is no reason why these ageless people cannot live for many years.

The Bible states, before the great flood, people lived as long as 900 years. We laugh this off by saying that these people measured their years in an entirely different way than we do, but how can we be sure of that? It is quite possible that these people knew how to eat and live to keep their arteries in perfect working order. Health is an orderly, harmonious functioning of the body, and this state of harmony continues as long as the heart, arteries and blood do their work effectively.

When we speak of people being old, we mean only one thing – they didn't know how to eat and live to keep their arteries unobstructed and healthy. When these damaged arteries are not doing their work correctly the blood can't get into the brain, and people become senile, forgetful and often lapse into a second childhood. They are dying a slow death because of it.

Smile at each other, smile at your wife, smile at your husband, smile at your children, smile at each other – it doesn't matter who it is – and that will help you grow in greater love for each other. – Mother Teresa

Eat Healthy – Live Healthy – Live Long

When we fast for a 24 to 36 hour period, or from 3 to 10 days, all the Vital Force in the body is used for internal purification . . . which includes purification of the arteries in the body. That is why after a 10 day fast there will be a feeling of lightness in the body, the mind will become keener, more alert and the memory will improve. The craving for physical activity will often become intense. Fasting helps to keep the arteries clean, healthy, elastic and more youthful.

I must reiterate the importance of a thorough check of the urine. During the 10 day fast, it should be bottled each morning and saved for observation. The faster will note a tremendous amount of heavy foreign substances that have been eliminated from the body, particularly the heavy mucus toxins that appear in the urine.

In my opinion, we can add years to our hearts with a systematic program of fasting, coupled with The Bragg Healthy Lifestyle program of natural food which reduces the waxy cholesterol that clogs arteries. We must think of our arteries as the key to life if we want to win the greatest battle in life – staying alive on this earth. When you stuff yourself on high-fat meals day after day you are bound to accumulate toxins, cholesterol and obstructions. Retribution is bound to come. Americans are the biggest eaters of fat in the world. Consequently we lead the world in cardiovascular diseases.

This is one reason that I believe in the No Breakfast Plan. I have known many young, healthy men and women who made it a habit every morning to eat a so-called hearty breakfast of ham and eggs or bacon and eggs, buttered toast, fried potatoes and coffee loaded with cream. Many of these supposedly healthy people were stricken with heart attacks or strokes that either killed them or made them invalids for the rest of their lives.

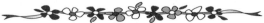

To fare well implies partaking of foods which do not disagree with body or mind. Hence only those who fare well live temperately. – Socrates

The Heart and Circulatory System

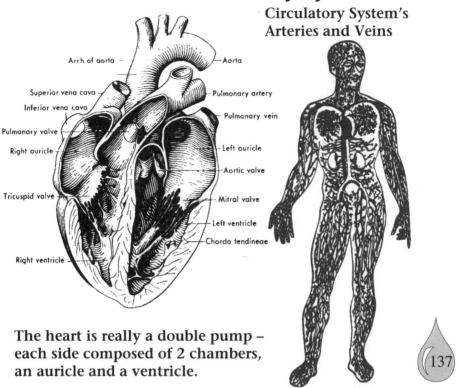

Circulatory System's
Arteries and Veins

Arch of aorta

Aorta

Superior vena cava

Pulmonary artery

Inferior vena cava

Pulmonary vein

Pulmonary valve

Right auricle

Left auricle

Aortic valve

Tricuspid valve

Mitral valve

Left ventricle

Chorda tendineae

Right ventricle

**The heart is really a double pump –
each side composed of 2 chambers,
an auricle and a ventricle.**

137

You cannot eat any food simply because you think it agrees with you! You won't make this mistake if you know about the physiology of the body and about nutrition; eating is a science, which means it's more than tickling the palate. Eating is a serious function, particularly if you want to keep your arteries clean, unobstructed and unblocked and healthy for life.

Before you go on the program that I have outlined in this book, get a thorough physical examination by a good health doctor. Have him acquaint you with the condition of your heart, arteries and blood. Know your blood pressures, pulse and blood cholesterol (chart page 138) and then follow this healthy lifestyle for a year. Then return to your doctor for an examination again. I believe your doctor will say you have made a miraculous transformation in your body in one short year. Again, remember you are only as young as your arteries and cardiovascular system – your river of life.

Healthy Heart Habits for a Long, Vital Life

Remember, organic live foods make live people; you are what you eat, drink, breathe, think and do, so eat a low-fat, low-sugar, high-fiber diet of natural whole grains, sprouts, fresh salad greens, vegetables, fruits, raw seeds, nuts, juices and chemical-free, pure distilled water.

Earn your food with daily exercise, for regular exercise improves your health, stamina, flexibility and endurance, and helps open the cardiovascular system. Only 45 minutes a day can do miracles for your mind and body. You become revitalized with new zest for living.

We are made of tubes. To help keep them clean and open, make a mixture using ½ raw oat bran and ½ psyllium husk powder and add 1 to 3 tsp daily to juices, pep drinks, herb teas, soups, hot cereals, foods, etc. Also I take 1 cayenne capsule (40,000 HU) daily with meals.

Another way to guard against clogged tubes daily is add 2 Tbsp soy lecithin granules (fat emulsifier) to beverages, veggies, soups, etc.

Take 50 to 100 mgs regular-released niacin (B-3) with one meal daily to help cleanse and open the cardiovascular system. Skin flushing may occur, nothing to worry about as it shows it's working! After cholesterol level reaches 180 or lower, take 1 to 2 niacin weekly.

Your heart needs a healthy balance of nutrients, so take a natural multi vitamin-mineral food supplement with extra vitamin E (mixed tocopherols), vitamin C, magnesium orotate, selenium, zinc, beta carotene and the amino acid L-Carnitine–these are your heart's super helpers! It's also wise to take bromelain and a multi-digestive enzyme with each meal – it aids digestion, assimilation and elimination.

Many with sleep problems use Melatonin or its tea for results.

Also use the amazing antioxidants pycnogenol or grape seed extract or SOD (super oxide dismutase). They help flush out dangerous free radicals that can cause havoc with your cardiovascular pipes and general health. Latest research shows extra benefits, promotes longevity, slows ageing, fights toxins, arthritis and its stiffness, swelling and pain, and helps prevent cataracts, jet lag, exhaustion and disease.

Count your blessings daily while you do your 30 to 40 minute brisk walk and exercises with these affirmations – health! strength! youth! vitality! peace! laughter! humility! understanding! forgiveness! joy! and love for eternity!– and soon all these qualities will come flooding and bouncing into your life. With blessings of super health, peace and love to you, our dear friends – our readers. – Patricia Bragg

Recommended Blood Chemistry Values
• Total Cholesterol: 180 mg/dl or less; 150 mg/dl or less is optimal
• Total Cholesterol, Childhood Years: 140 mg/dl or less
• HDL Cholesterol: Men, 50 mg/dl or more; Women, 65 mg/dl or more
• HDL Cholesterol Ratio: 3.2 or less • Triglycerides: 100 mg/dl or less
• LDL Cholesterol: 100 mg/dl or less is optimal • Glucose: 80 -100 mg/dl

You Have
Nine Doctors
At Your Command

Mother Nature's 9 Doctors are ready to help you attain radiant, glorious health. They are all specialists in their particular fields of health building. They have had years and years of experience with thousands upon thousands of people. Their cumulative record is 100% perfect! They have never failed a patient. Patients have failed them, turned their backs on them and ignored them. But they are kind and understanding and, no matter how many times patients have failed them, they still stand ready to render perfect professional service. They have but one prescription and that is elixir of life! They are the kindest Doctors in the whole universe! They are anxious and willing to help everyone who comes to them for Higher Health. Their professional services are available to all – the young, the old, the rich and the poor. They perform no operations except bloodless ones. They give no drugs, not even any so-called "wonder drugs."

139

You are all familiar with these 9 wonderful life-changing Doctors – we all need them. I want you to call on these 9 Doctors frequently. They are so eager to help you help yourself to supreme health, youthfulness, longevity and agelessness! This is the Highest Health you can have; you should have it your entire long life!

These wonderful Doctors will never, ever fail you. They want to be your personal care givers and also your friends. It gives me a most secure feeling that I have at my command, every day, the world's great Doctors and it's my pleasure to introduce you to them. From this day on, please feel free to call upon them. First, I want you to meet the Father of them all, the most eminent and the greatest healer and giver of life to everything on the face of this earth . . . Doctor Sunshine.

The laws of health are inexorable; we see people going down and out in their prime of life because no attention is paid to them! – Paul C. Bragg

KEEP HEALTHY & YOUTHFUL BIOLOGICALLY WITH EXERCISE & GOOD NUTRITION

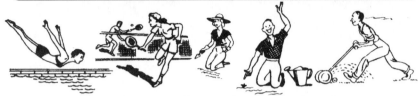

Always remember you have the following important reasons for following The Bragg Healthy Lifestyle:

- The ironclad laws of Mother Nature and God.
- Your common sense, which tells you that you are doing right.
- Your aim to make your health better and your life longer.
- Your resolve to prevent illness so that you may enjoy life.
- Make an art of healthy living; you will be youthful at any age.
- You will retain your faculties and be hale, hearty, active and useful far beyond the ordinary length of years.
- You will also possess superior mental and physical powers!

WANTED – For Robbing Health & Life

KILLER Saturated Fats	CHOKER Hydrogenated Fats
CLOGGER Salt	DEADEYED Devitalized Foods
DOPEY Caffeine	HARD WATER Inorganic Minerals
PLUGGER Frying Pan	JERKY Turbulent Emotions
DEATH-DEALER Drugs	CRAZY Alcohol
GREASY Overweight	SMOKY Tobacco
HOGGY Overeating	LOAFER Laziness

What Wise Men Say

Wisdom does not show itself so much in precept as in life – a firmness of mind and mastery of appetite. – Seneca

Govern well thy appetite, lest Sin surprise thee, & her black attendant, Death. – Milton

Our prayers should be for a sound mind in a healthy body. – Juvenal

I saw few die of hunger – of eating, a hundred thousand. – Ben Franklin

Health consists of temperance alone. – Pope

Health is…a blessing that money cannot buy. – Izaak Walton

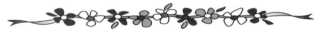

The natural healing force within us is the greatest force in getting well.
– Hippocrates, Father of Medicine

Of all the knowledge, that most worth having is the knowledge about health! The first requisite of a good life is to be a healthy person. – Herbert Spencer

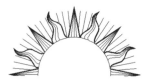

Chapter 19

Doctor Sunshine

Doctor Sunshine's specialty is heliotherapy and his great prescription is solar energy. Each tiny blade of grass, every vine, tree, bush, flower, fruit and vegetable draws its life from solar energy. All living things on earth depend on solar energy for their very existence. This earth would be a barren, frigid place if it were not for the magic rays of the sun. The sun gives us light and were it not for sunshine, there would be no you or me. The earth would be in everlasting darkness.

Human beings were never meant to have pale skins, not even the fair northern races. Man's skin should be lightly tanned by the sun and should take on a darker pigment according to his original skin tone. It has been found that even fair, red-headed people will tan. Pigmentation is a sign that solar energy has been transformed into human energy. By enjoying the early morning or late afternoon gentle sunshine man can gain more health, vitality and happiness. The people who are indoors too long have sallow-looking skin. This is why many women hide sun-starved skins with makeup.

141

The person who is starved of the vital rays of the sun has a half-dead look. He is actually dying for the want of solar energy! Weak, ailing and anemic people are all sun-starved and – in my opinion – many people are sick simply because they are starving for gentle sunshine.

The sunshine's gentle rays have powerful germicidal properties. As the skin gathers these gentle rays, it stores up enormous amounts of this germ-killing energy. The sun provides one of the finest remedies for the nervous person who is filled with anxiety, worry and frustration.

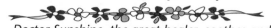

Doctor Sunshine, the great healer, soothes and
sparkles your body inside and outside! – Paul C. Bragg

Sunshine Brings Peace, Relaxation to Nerves

When nervous people lie in the sunshine, its soothing, gentle rays give them what their nerves and body are crying out for – relaxation! Sunshine is a health tonic and a Great Healer! As you bask in the warm sunshine, millions of nerve endings absorb the solar energy and transform and store them into more Vital Force for your nerves and body.

Perform this experiment to determine the value of sunshine in the matter of life and death. Find a beautiful patch of lawn where the grass is like a green carpet. Cover up a small space of that beautiful lawn with a small piece of wood or metal. Day by day you will notice that the beautiful grass that was so full of plant blood, or chlorophyll, will start to fade and turn a sickly yellow. Then the tragedy happens. It withers and dies - death from sun starvation! The same thing happens in your body without the life giving rays of the sun. This also happens when you fail to eat an abundance of sun-grown foods such as ripe, organic fruits and vegetables.

142

We must have the direct rays of the sun on our bodies and our diet must contain 60% or more of food that has been ripened by the sun's rays. When we eat fresh fruits and vegetables we absorb the blood of the plant – the rich, nourishing chlorophyll. Chlorophyll is the solar energy that the plant has absorbed from the sun, the richest and most nourishing food you can put into your body. "Chlorophyll is liquid sunshine." Green plants alone possess the secret of how to capture this powerful solar energy and pass it on to man and every other living creature.

When you put sunshine on the outside of your body and 60% to 70% raw fruits and vegetables in your daily diet, you are going to glow with radiant health! But these are powerful and must be taken in small doses at the start, because your sun-starved body has to slowly get used to these cleansing, solar-powered foods.

The law, "Whatsoever a man sows that he shall also reap," is inscribed in flaming letters upon the portal of Eternity, and none can deny it, none can cheat it, none can escape it. –James Allen

Gentle Sun Rays are Soothing and Best

When you take your first sunbath, start with short time periods until you can condition your body to longer exposure. The best time for a beginner to start taking gentle sunbaths is in the early morning sunshine. Or you may sunbathe in the late afternoon gentle sunshine. Five to ten minutes on the nude body is sufficient at first. Avoid the burning rays between 11 am and 3 pm. The best cool rays of the sun are in the early morning.

The same caution should be taken in eating sun ripened foods – the raw fruits and vegetables. The average person who has been eating mainly cooked foods will find that if great amounts of raw fruit and vegetables are suddenly put into the body they can cause a reaction. It's wiser to add more sun-grown foods to the diet gradually. Overdoses of solar energy, both on the outside and the inside of the body, are not good. Regarding exposure to the sun, it's quite necessary to use good judgment and always proceed with caution.

At this point I must add a personal touch. At 16 years of age I had been sentenced to death with deadly tuberculosis. The greatest doctors in the United States declared me "Hopeless! Incurable!" By the Grace of God I was led to Dr. August Rollier of Leysen, Switzerland, the greatest living authority on Heliotherapy (Sun Cure). High in the Alps, Dr. Rollier exposed my sick, wasted body to the healing rays of the sun and fed me an abundance of sun-grown foods. Presto! A miracle happened! In 2 short years I was transformed from a bed-ridden invalid to a strong, healthy, young man.

I am way over 85 years young and I am still a powerful and healthy man. Through all of these long years I have kept the glorious light of the sun's gentle rays on my body. I regained my health through the gentle healing of "Doctor Healing Sunshine." He helped save my life and that is why I love God's own precious sunshine.

Every man is the builder of a temple called his body. We are all sculptors and painters, and our material is our own flesh and blood and bones. Any nobleness begins at once to refine a man's features, any meanness or sensuality to imbrute them. – Henry David Thoreau

I Love Being With Doctor Sunshine

Patricia and I love the great sunshine state and have a home in the Santa Monica mountains so we can enjoy the mountain sunshine. We have a modest home in the California Desert, where the sun shines 354 days a year, and a cottage and our organic veggie garden and flowers in Santa Barbara near our office, and a place in Hawaii at Diamond Head near our free exercise class (page iii). We are great beach walkers and spend hours, in winter and summer, on the sun drenched beaches of Hawaii, Florida, France, Australia and New Zealand while on our Health Crusades. Seek the gentle sunshine and health follows by leaps and bounds.

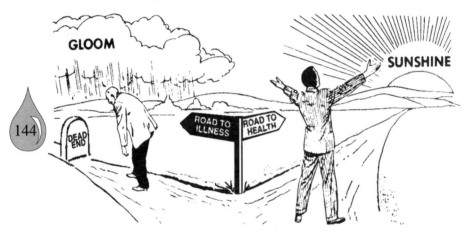

The choice of which road to take is up to the individual. He alone can decide whether he wants to reach a dead end or live a healthy lifestyle for a long, healthy, happy, active life. – Paul C. Bragg

Deprivation of food at first brings a sensation of hunger, occasionally some nervous stimulation – but it also determines certain hidden phenomena which are more important. The sugar of the liver and the fat of the subcutaneous deposits are mobilized, as are the proteins of the muscles and glands. All the organs sacrifice their own substances in order to maintain blood, heart and brain in a normal condition. Fasting purifies and profoundly modifies our tissues.
– Dr. Alexis Carrel, Nobel Prize winner, author of *Man, the Unknown*

The secret of longevity is eating intelligently. – Gayelord Hauser

Always do what is right – despite any public opinions.

Chapter 20

Doctor Fresh Air

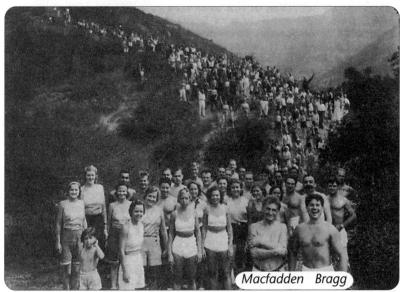

Macfadden   Bragg

A thousand Happy Bragg Health Students Enjoying Hiking, Exercise and Fresh Air on The Trail to Mt. Hollywood, California. Summer, 1932. In the left foreground is Bernarr Macfadden, Father and Founder of the Physical Culture Movement and Publisher of popular Physical Culture Magazine and, to the right, Paul C. Bragg, Health Crusader and Life Extension Specialist. These Health Pioneers enjoyed leading Health and Fitness Crusades across America.

Doctor Fresh Air is a health specialist, and his greatest prescription for you is to "Breathe Deeply of God's Pure Fresh Air." The first thing we do when we are born is take a long, deep breath and the last thing we do is take a last gasp before we stop breathing. Between birth and death, life is completely maintained by breathing.

Doctor Fresh Air wants you to have a long active life and he feels, as a specialist, that you will if you follow his simple instructions and breathe deeply. You must always be conscious that, with every breath you take, you are bringing into your body the Breath of God . . . which is life-giving oxygen. People who fail to obey this doctor's orders about getting plenty of fresh air every day and night are inviting some severe complications.

The Lord God formed man of the dust of the ground, and breathed into his nostrils the breath of life; and man became a living soul. – Genesis 2:7

145

Our Body is a Breathing Machine

Let us examine very closely the function of breathing. First, it is invisible food. It is the only food that we cannot be deprived of for over 7 minutes or death will take us. We not only receive life-giving oxygen that is so necessary to every cell in our bodies from the air, but when we breathe, oxygen is carried by the blood to the lungs where a great miracle takes place. There the life-giving oxygen is exchanged for deadly carbon dioxide, in which form many of the deadly toxins of the body are released. In other words, we create toxic poisons in our body during the very process of living. These are collected by the blood as it circulates and, after the blood brings carbon dioxide to the lungs, it's expelled as the new life-giving oxygen enters. Carbon dioxide is also burned up through the process of metabolism and during the creation and destruction of the cells of the body.

If a person doesn't get enough fresh air – or if they are a shallow breather – and the oxygen intake doesn't equal the outgo of carbon dioxide, then these toxic poisons build up within the body structure. This can result in serious physical problems as the retained carbon dioxide can concentrate in other parts of the body to cause intense physical suffering.

Enervation, the lack of nerve energy, can lower the Vital Force so much that the body's great bellows – the lungs – cannot pump in enough air to flush the carbon dioxide out of the body. See how important it is that you not only breathe fresh air, but always be conscious of the fact that you must breathe deeply in and out.

We are air machines. Oxygen not only purifies the body, but is also one of the great energizers of the human body. We are air pressure machines. We live at the bottom of an atmospheric ocean approximately 70 miles deep. This air pressure is 14 pounds per square inch. Between the inhalation and the exhalation of a breath, a vacuum is formed. As long as we continue to have this rhythmical intake and output of oxygen, we will live. We can go without food for 30 days and more and still survive but we can go without air only a few minutes.

Deep Breathers Live Longer

Air is one of the important energizers of the human body. The more deeply you breathe pure air, the better your chances are for extending your life on this earth. For over 75 years, I have done extensive research on long-lived people and I've discovered one common denominator among them all. They are deep breathers. I have found that the deeper, therefore fewer breaths a person takes in one minute, the longer they live. Most rapid breathers are the short-lived people.

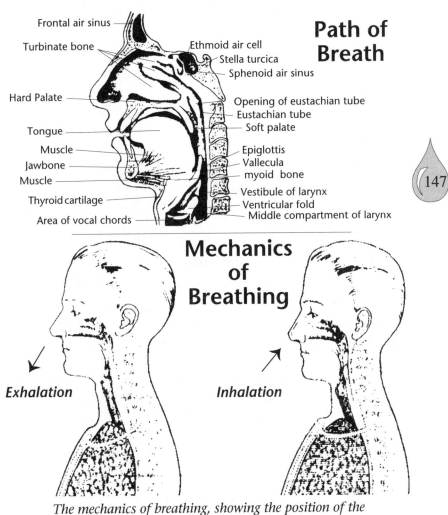

Path of Breath

- Frontal air sinus
- Turbinate bone
- Ethmoid air cell
- Stella turcica
- Sphenoid air sinus
- Hard Palate
- Opening of eustachian tube
- Eustachian tube
- Soft palate
- Tongue
- Muscle
- Epiglottis
- Jawbone
- Vallecula
- Muscle
- myoid bone
- Thyroid cartilage
- Vestibule of larynx
- Ventricular fold
- Area of vocal chords
- Middle compartment of larynx

147

Mechanics of Breathing

Exhalation

Inhalation

The mechanics of breathing, showing the position of the diaphragm and ribs at exhalation and at inhalation

Breathing is the greatest pleasure in life. – Papini

Yes, rapid breathing humans shorten their lives and this also applies to the animal world. Rabbits, guinea pigs and all kinds of rodents are rapid breathers. They are the shortest-lived animals. For years I have made it a practice when I first get up in the morning to do my long, slow, deep breathing exercises and practice them several times throughout the day.

India's Holy Men Practice Deep, Slow Breathing

On my expeditions to India I found holy men at secluded retreats who had devoted their lives to building a physically powerful body as an instrument for high spiritual advancement. They spent many hours daily in the practice of rhythmic, long, slow, deep breathing. These holy men of India were in utterly fantastic physical condition because the deep breathing of fresh air kept their skin and muscle tone ageless! I met a holy man in the foothills of the Himalaya Mountains who told me that he was, at that time, 126 years old! This man had no reason to lie to me because his whole life was spent in getting closer to God. It was he who taught me the system which I teach all over the world known as "Super Power Breathing." I do not have sufficient space in this book to detail the full program that this holy man taught me, but do read our book *Bragg Super Power Breathing*.

To go into further detail in describing this holy man physically, he had perfect vision and he had a beautiful head of hair with not one gray hair in it. He had all his teeth and he possessed the endurance and stamina of an athlete. He spoke seven languages fluently. He was one of the most amazing men that I have ever met in my life! When I asked him to what he owed his great strength and mentality, his answer was, "I have made a lifelong practice of breathing deeply and practicing faithfully all of my breathing exercises daily."

As a man, I don't like to guess the age of any woman. But while I was on a trip to India I met a woman whose age I guessed to be around 50. I was amazed when she told me she was 86! She was beautiful with no signs of ageing. When I asked her the secret of her beauty and her agelessness, I got the same answer I did from the holy man. This beautiful woman was totally aware of the importance of deep breathing for her health.

You must have noticed children playing and running, jumping rope, roller skating and bicycling. While they are doing these activities, they are breathing in large amounts of oxygen, and that is what we must keep in mind. We must keep active and take long, brisk walks and cultivate the habit of deep breathing. When I find people living sedentary lives, no longer getting vigorous exercise, I know that they are shortening their lives.

Deep Breathing – Secret of Endurance

A friend of mine for many years was Amos Stagg, the famous football and athletic coach. Mr. Stagg lived to be over 100 years of age. I once asked him his secret of long life and his answer was, "I have all of my life indulged in running and other vigorous exercises that forced large amounts of oxygen into my body."

I had another friend in New York, James Hocking, who was one of the greatest long distance walking champions America has ever had. I asked Mr. Hocking, on his hundredth birthday the secret of his long active life and super health. His answer was "I have always walked vigorously and breathed deeply." So you see, oxygen is a detoxifier. It is like fasting, it continually helps remove the poisons from the body.

I not only practice deep breathing personally, but I also believe that people should expose their bodies to a current of freely moving air. Air baths are important to good health. You should sleep with your windows wide open and with a cross ventilation of air moving across your bed. I find that I sleep better and have a deeper night's rest if I don't wear sleeping garments and when I do, I wear light cotton or silk. Under the covers it's warm and if you pile on extra sleeping garments you close off the skin from its supply of oxygen.

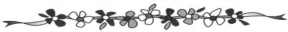

The quality of the blood depends largely upon its oxygenation in the lungs.

Americans Are Becoming Lazy Sitters

If you sit for hours, you must compensate for this inactivity because it's then that your breathing slows down. If your occupation requires a lot of sitting, you should compensate with outdoor walking and physical activities. You will find that you can solve most of your problems during a brisk 2 mile hike in the fresh air. I do this and it helps me. I believe that after the evening meal everyone should make a practice of taking a walk, even if it has to be up and down your driveway or hall.

Today we are a society of sitters! We sit at our desks, the movies, concerts, sports events and watching television. We are air and oxygen-starved. We can't get the toxic carbon dioxide out of our bodies, so we are full of aches and pains and prone to premature ageing. This is all because we are too lazy and too indifferent about being active, vigorous people! Everywhere you look you will see mostly overweight, unhealthy, exhausted people. Many of their problems are due to lack of oxygen. That's why it's so important to fast; because it helps to clean up any stored carbon dioxide that failed to leave your body through deep breathing.

So when you are fasting, and feel up to it – enjoy a short walk. Between fasts, make it a part of your life to be an active person. This means getting out in the fresh air to enjoy brisk walking, hiking, running, swimming, tennis, etc. Join a gym and try dancing, also. You must not allow carbon dioxide to pile up in your body! This brings serious consequences.

Pray for wisdom in your daily living, for more faith and for more patience with yourself and others before you pray for just things.

Living under conditions of modern life, it is important to bear in mind that the preparation and refinement of food products either entirely eliminates or in part destroys the vital elements in the original material.
– United States Department of Agriculture

You can increase the oxygen currents of nerve force with the breath and send it to heal parts of your body. – Paul C. Bragg

Deep Breathing Builds Powerful Body

So, along with your fasting program, make it a point every day of your life to have a brisk 2 to 5 mile walk and, during that walk, breathe deeply. Every time you think of it during your waking hours, you must take long, slow, deep breaths. Remember what I told you – the more long, slow, deep breaths you take, the longer you will live. When you combine deep breathing with fasting you are adding years to your life! You are building energy and vitality. You are going to break free of many miseries by fasting and deep breathing. Remind yourself every day that Doctor Fresh Air is your constant friend.

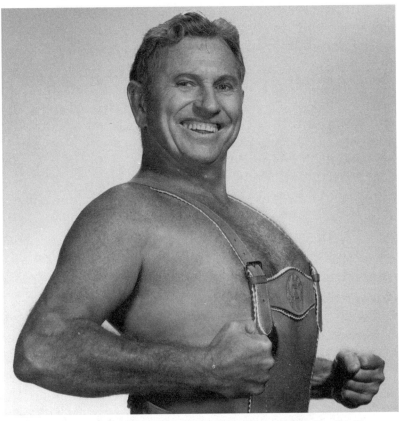

151

The Bragg System of *Super Power Breathing* Built Bragg a Powerful, Healthy Body. Do read the book *Super Power Breathing*. See back pages for booklist.

The strongest principle of growth lies in the human choice. – George Elliot

Fluorine is a Deadly Poison

Millions of innocent people have been brainwashed by the aluminum companies to erroneously believe that adding sodium fluoride (their waste by-product) to our drinking water will reduce tooth decay in our children. Americans get sodium fluoride in their drinking water without thinking about it. A chemical cousin of sodium, fluorine in high doses is used as a rat and roach killer and a deadly pesticide.

Yet this deadly sodium fluoride, injected virtually by government edict into drinking water in the proportion of 1.2 parts per million (PPM), has been declared by the US Public Health Service to be "safe for all human consumption." Every chemist knows that such "absolute safety" is not only unattainable, but a total illusion!

Keep Toxic Fluoride Out of Your Water!

152

Most water Americans drink has fluoride in it, including tap, bottled and canned drinks and foods! Now, the ADA (American Dental Association) is insisting that the FDA mandate the addition of fluoride to all bottled waters! Defend your right to drink pure, nonfluoridated tap and bottled waters! Challenge and stop local and state water fluoridation policies! Call, write, fax or e-mail all your state officials and Congresspeople and send them a copy of this book.

Check the Following Web Sites for Fluoride Updates:

- www.bragg.com   • www.citizens.org
- www.sonic.net/~kryptox/fluoride.htm
- www.cadvision.com/fluoride/index.htm
- emporium.turnpike.net/P/PDHA/fluoride/fluor.htm
- www.garynull.com/documents/fluoridation.htm

These 11 Associations Stopped Endorsing Water Fluoridation in 1996

- *American Heart Assoc.* • *American Academy of Allergy & Immunology*
- *American Cancer Society* • *Chronic Fatigue Syndrome Action Network*
- *American Diabetes Assoc.* • *National Institute of Law Municipal Officers*
- *American Chiropractic Assoc.* • *American Civil Liberties Union* • *Soc. of Toxicology*
- *National Kidney Foundation*   • *American Psychiatric Association*

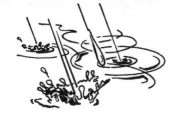

Chapter 21

Doctor Pure Water

The Water You Drink Can Make or Break Your Health!

Doctor Pure Water is a vitally important healer and splendid friend. Water is involved in nearly every body process (page 155). I have thoroughly explained the importance of drinking distilled water, the best for your health, in another part of this book. Water makes up about 70% of your body, so you need a continuous replacement to keep your water level normal and healthy. Optimum is 8 to 10 glasses daily. When you eat fruits and vegetables you are also adding their liquids (distilled by nature) to your diet.

There's so many health benefits from water you can enjoy. A good warm bath is a tonic and a relaxer which soothes irritated nerves and quiets emotions. Every day of the year in the United States people enjoy swimming in water at the seashore, in lakes, rivers, streams and swimming pools. Swimming is one of the best exercises anyone can perform. It puts no strain on the joints or the heart. Swim as often as you can. If you can't swim, go to a professional who can teach you how to swim. You will never regret it because it is one of the most relaxing, but exhilarating of exercises. It can be enjoyed regardless of age. Don't fear it! Learn to love it.

Water therapies have been used for man's miseries since the beginning of time. In my world travels I have found many different types of therapies. It's been proven that the ancient civilizations of the Egyptians, Assyrians, Hebrews, Persians, Greeks, Hindus, Chinese and other cultures, including Native American Indians, have used water therapies for the relief of human ailments.

153

The noblest of the elements is water. – Pindar

Most Ancient Healers Used Water Therapy

400 years before the birth of Christ, on the Greek island of Cos in the Aegean Sea, Hippocrates, the father of medicine developed a complete system of water treatments. His records state that a cold bath followed by a hot bath and a massage improves the circulation. We agree with this! The cold then hot bath followed by a coarse friction rub is one of the best circulation builders.

I have visited great health (water) spas around the world. For years we had a home in Desert Hot Springs, California, so we could enjoy their healing waters. It's located directly on the San Andreas fault where many earthquakes originate. Under this fault there is a great river of hot mineral water. Wells are piped down to this underground river and the hot mineral water is brought to the spas. People from all over the world come to Desert Hot Springs to bathe in its soothing mineral water.

I do not regard hot mineral water as a cure for any human ailment. But I believe that hot water, particularly at 104°, is a purifier and a detoxifier that increases the body's circulation. This is why I recommend a hot Epsom salts or apple cider vinegar bath (1 cup) as a detoxifier and relaxer. It should be taken in water anywhere from 98° to 104°. You should remain in this bath 10 minutes and no more. The special bath can be a very important part of your health program. Usually it's best not to take a hot bath during your fasts – but warm water is O.K.

Always remember that clean, pure water inside and outside is the best to use. It's one of Mother Nature's wonderful ways of building a healthy body. Distilled water is the best for drinking and all food uses.

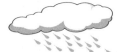 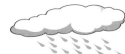 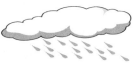

The Health Miracles of Water

To the days of the aged it addeth length;
To the might of the strong it addeth strength;
It freshens the heart, it brightens the sight;
'Tis like quaffing a goblet of morning light.

Water is More Important than Food

More than 70% of the human body is water. The bones in your body are even 30% water. To lose a tenth of your body's water supply is dangerous, and to lose a fifth can be fatal. Losing lesser amounts disturbs body functions and impairs chemical and physical processes necessary to good health. Yet the body itself can take lots of punishment. Half your proteins and almost all of your fat and glycogen can be lost without causing death. Only that important 70% of your body – water – requires that it be kept at a consistently high level.

A practical example of the body's demand for water can be drawn from mountain climbing histories. In their assault on the Himalayas, men working and climbing in high altitudes cut down on the weight they carried in an attempt to conserve body energy. None were notably successful until a team conquering Mount Everest scientifically considered the effect of the altitude on the body's water metabolism. These men increased their fuel load in order to melt snow and ice into water. They were assured of an average of 6 pints of water daily per person, much more than any previous teams had considered as adequate rations. While water was not the sole contributing factor to their success, it was recognized as helping to prevent the fatigue experienced by former teams during their final assaults. The rest of us may not need water for anything as demanding as climbing the Himalayas, but this serves as an example of how important water – or the lack of it – in our diets can be.

Water is the Key to All Body Functions!

- Heart
- Circulation
- Digestion
- Bones & Joints
- Muscles
- Metabolism
- Assimilation
- Elimination
- Sex
- Glands
- Nerves
- Energy

The power of pure water is the vital chemistry of life!

How Our Body Uses Water

Almost every fluid connected with life and living things is based on water. Protoplasm (the substance regarded as the physical basis of life) cannot exist without water. Nor can a blade of grass, a cactus, an insect, a bird or a fish, etc. Dry out a living cell and it will stop working. It must have liquid to survive and live!

Human cells are the very same. Even food is brought to them via fluid in the form of blood. There are about 9 pints of blood in your body. After food is consumed by the cells, the waste is carried away in a water-based liquid, your urine. Even oxygen cannot be absorbed by your lungs except through a moist surface. The same is true of the waste by-product of oxygen, carbon dioxide.

Water is Necessary For Digestion

Food can't be digested without water. There is an actual chemical process that goes on in your body that's known as "hydrolysis." It involves changing proteins, starches and fats into foods that various cells require in order to work properly. But water is also necessary to stimulate gastric glands in the stomach. In the intestines it helps facilitate the absorption of solids and the most important excretion of wastes.

Water is important to digestion. It begins with the intake of food at the mouth. Here the fluid known as saliva – which is 99.5% water – begins the digestion of carbohydrates. The gastric juices we've mentioned earlier are 90% water – they work on the food passed on to the stomach from the mouth. The food, now fairly liquid, is next passed to the duodenum, or upper section of the small intestine, where enzymes, the liver secretions and the pancreas (90% water) finish digestion of food.

Food is passed through the intestines and absorbed through the intestinal walls in a watery state. The largest portion of this absorption occurs in the colon. Diarrhea results from unabsorbed water which is passed as waste. This is a dangerous situation for infants who, because of their size have only a small supply of water. This can result in dehydration, bad digestion and even death.

Somewhere between 7 and 11 quarts of water are needed just for proper digestion. Breaking this down, it comes to 3 pints of saliva, a couple of quarts of gastric juice, plus an equivalent amount of bile and other glandular and intestinal secretions. Fortunately, the body is thrifty and most of this moisture is absorbed and recycled. Its first job after being absorbed is to transfer the newly digested foods to the cells through the bloodstream where the blood cells themselves use and reuse the water in their own process of living.

Water is Vital in Removing Body Waste

Water plays an important role in the excretion of waste through the intestine. The other forms of soluble waste also rely on water. The kidneys, bladder, skin and lungs all depend heavily on water to rid themselves of any body poisons and excretions on a regular basis.

The lung walls are composed of tiny air sacs that, in order to function properly during the intake of oxygen and the expulsion of carbon dioxide, must be moist. The linings of the nose, throat, trachea and bronchial tubes are also always moist – or should be. Because of all this contact with air, the body loses about a pint of water every day solely through exhalation. When the air is very dry, even more moisture is lost. Many people replace this moisture by using a vaporizer in their homes.

A large quantity of water can be lost through the skin. Here water is used as a vehicle for waste. The kidneys use water rapidly, but the amount they use depends on the quantity of fluid you drink. For every quart of water passed through the kidneys, 1½ ounces of waste are carried in it. This is normal, but water (as urine) never falls below a level of a little more than a half of a pint. Kidneys never stop working and constantly demand water, even when none is available. The body is then forced to supply it through dehydration to live. All of these functions occur without any chemical transformation of the water. Water always remains water.

A strong body makes a strong mind. – Thomas Jefferson, 3rd U.S. President

Blood Plasma is 90% Water

Sure, blood is thicker than water . . . but only by about 10%! Blood plasma is 90% water which permits it to circulate through the body freely. It carries all sorts of nutrients and gases, inorganic salts and products, wastes and items needed for body functions, activity and growth.

Everything used by body cells is transported by plasma, including the material the cell is made from. Anything made by these same cells which is needed in other parts of the body – or to be excreted – is carried by the same plasma. Yet plasma remains fairly identical in composition at all times throughout the body. As it absorbs foods and fuels from the digestive and respiratory processes, it has the same substances taken from it by body tissues, including the kidneys and lungs. If this important balance is to be always healthy and maintained, it's vitally important to have sufficient water for your blood.

Water Helps Keeps You Cool and Healthy

Automobiles have water in their radiators to help cool their engines. It's much the same with the human body. The reason is that water absorbs heat readily. In living organisms, where constant internal temperatures are often critical, water acts as a vital and efficient coolant. The human body has a constant temperature level. Measured orally, this is 98.6° F. It shouldn't vary much despite the climate or temperature surrounding the body.

This internal temperature is controlled by external skin evaporation to a large degree. Just about a fourth of the heat created by the processing of oxygen and food by the body is eliminated through normal perspiration and the process of breathing. But under exceptionally dry conditions, the body can lose up to a quart of water an hour through the sweating process alone. Obviously, this water has to be replaced or other functions of the body are impaired. When it's cold, the body can actually

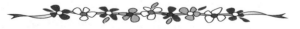

Miracles can happen every day through guidance and prayer! – Patricia Bragg

cease perspiring and water is further withdrawn into the tissues. The evaporation of water from skin surfaces results in cooling – Mother Nature's air conditioning and fevers are in a way related. When you sweat and feel hot, perhaps you have a temperature. When your skin is dry and you feel chills, perhaps your body temperature has dipped. These often are signs of illness.

In humid weather, evaporation is more difficult. So we feel hotter though we're sweating. Our body has a harder time cooling off and ends up working harder to keep it cool. Researchers have found that the average man, doing nothing, will lose about 23 ounces of fluid via the lungs and skin on a day that has normal humidity. A long distance runner, on the other hand, will lose as much as 8 pounds. Football players can shed almost 14 pounds of water in about an hour's time!

Because the body is more than 70% water, and because excretory processes depend so much on it, water is easy to lose. Many so-called diets are based on lower water consumption or increasing water loss. This can be very dangerous, especially if practiced over a period of time. Fatigue is one of the first signs of water deficiency. It should be heeded by drinking lots of water!

Water – The Body's Vital Lubricant

The body, in its own way, is greased and oiled automatically. The body's basic lubricant is water. It permits organs to slide against each other – such as when you bend down. It helps the bones to move in their joints. You couldn't bend a knee or elbow without it. Also, it acts as a shock-absorbing agent to ward off injury from blows. Applied hydraulically in various parts of the body, it is used to build and hold pressures. The eyeball is a good example of this particular function of water. Muscle tone cannot be maintained without adequate water, for the muscles are ¾ water. This is another reason why fatigue hits the dehydrated body.

Water flows through every single part of your body, cleansing and nourishing it. But the wrong kind of water – with inorganic minerals, harmful toxins, chemicals and other contaminants can pollute, clog and gradually turn every part of your body to stone. – Paul C. Bragg

The Body's Three Sources of Water

Your body has to obtain its water somehow. The first source is obvious. You drink water or a fluid containing it such as fruit juice, soup, beverages and the like. The second source is regular foods, which are mostly water. The delicious organic fruits and vegetables have the highest water content. Don't forget your body is about 70% water. A peach is almost all water – 90%. And even something as dry as a hard roll is ¼ water!

The third important source of water is metabolism. This is called metabolic water and it's made by the body from raw materials taken into the body. In other words, it's a chemically made water. It results from the cells' conversion of ingested food to cellular food. A perfect example of this type of water production is that biological water factory known as the camel. Now, the camel doesn't store water. It stores fat in the hump on its back. It also eats carbohydrates. In using these foods, the camel creates a great deal of water as a by-product and then uses the water in its body chemistry just as if it had drunk the water! Some insects are able to do this too, even though they eat exceptionally dry, low-water content foods. The average man consumes only about 2½ quarts of water a day by eating and drinking, but he uses up a full 2¾ quarts. The difference in this amount is his production of metabolic water.

Body Dehydration Causes Health Problems

When the body doesn't get enough water, it reacts and suffers. The precious secretions of important glands are drastically deprived. Saliva dries up and membranes dry out. We're thirsty. The body signals quickly that a drink of water is imperative! After losing more than a little water without replenishing the supply, other symptoms develop. Headaches, nervousness, inability to concentrate, digestive problems and lack of hunger are some of these. Water quickly alleviates these symptoms. American soldiers in the Arctic experienced personality problems when forced into low-water rations. To be deprived of water for just a few days can be deadly. The body needs 8 glasses of water a day to ensure health and survival. Do read our Water book.

The Apple Cider Vinegar Drink Helps The Urine to Keep a Healthy Acid Balance

The apple cider vinegar and distilled water drink taken the first thing in the morning aids in keeping the urine in a normal acid condition, for urine is naturally acidic. This shows that the kidneys are doing their duties efficiently, flushing out the body poisons. The drink consists of a 6 ounce glass of distilled water and 2 teaspoons equally of raw honey and Bragg's Raw Organic Apple Cider Vinegar, a natural unpasteurized, unfiltered vinegar that's aged in wood. (It's available in health stores worldwide!)

Go to any drugstore and purchase Squibb Nitrazine paper. Dip a small piece of this paper in your most recent urine sample immediately. There is a chart on the Nitrazine paper container for you to determine acidity. If it's yellow your urine is normal – that means it is acid. The chart will give you a truthful answer. Apples, grapes, cranberries, strawberries, cherries and raspberries will also keep your urine at normal acidity.

161

Distilled water is one of the world's best and purest waters! It is excellent for detoxification and fasting programs and for helping clean out all the cells, organs, and fluids of the body because it can help carry away so many harmful substances!

Water from chemically treated public water systems and even from wells and springs is likely to be loaded with poisonous chemicals and toxic trace elements. Depending upon the kind of piping that the water has been run through, the water in our homes and offices, schools, hospitals, etc., is likely to be overloaded with zinc (from old-fashioned galvanized pipes) or with copper and cadmium (from copper pipes). These trace elements are released in excessive quantity by the chemical action of the water on the metals of the pipes.

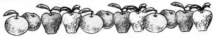

Knowing these teachings will mean true life and good health for you. – Proverbs 4:22

Health in a human being is the perfection of bodily organization, intellectual energy and moral power. – T.L. Nichols, M.D.

Pure Water is Essential For Health!

Yes, pure water is essential for health. You get it from the natural juices of vegetables, fruits and other foods, or from the water of high purity obtained by steam distillation which is the best method. Another effective method combines de-ionization and purification.

The body is constantly working for you, breaking down old bone and tissue cells and replacing them with new ones. As the body casts off the old minerals and other products of broken-down cells it must obtain new supplies of the essential elements for the new cells. Scientists are beginning to understand that various kinds of dental problems, many types of arthritis and some forms of hardening of the arteries are due to imbalances in the body's levels of calcium, phosphorus and magnesium. Disorders can also be caused by imbalances in the ratios of various minerals to each other.

Each healthy body requires a proper balance within itself of all the nutritive elements. It is just as bad for any individual to have too much of one item as it is to have too little of that one or of another one. It takes appropriate levels of phosphorus and magnesium to keep calcium in solution so it can be formed into new bone and teeth. Yet, there must not be too much of those nor too little calcium in the diet, or old bone will be taken away but new bone will not be formed.

In addition, we now know that diets which are unbalanced and inappropriate for a given individual can deplete the body of calcium, magnesium, potassium, and other major and minor elements. Diets which are high in meats, fish, eggs and grains or their products may provide unbalanced excesses of phosphorus. This will deplete calcium and magnesium from the bones and tissues of the body and cause them to be lost in the urine. A diet high in fats will tend to increase the uptake of phosphorus from the intestines relative to calcium and other basic minerals. Such a high-fat diet can produce losses of calcium, magnesium, and other basic minerals as a high-phosphorus diet does.

162

Pure water is the best drink for a wise man. – Henry David Thoreau

Mineral Imbalances are Dangerous

Diets excessively high in fruits or their juices may provide unbalanced excesses of potassium in the body and calcium and magnesium will again be lost from the body through the urine. The body likes a healthy balance! Deficiencies of calcium and magnesium, for example, can produce all kinds of problems in the body. They range from dental decay and osteoporosis to muscular cramping, hyperactivity, muscular twitching, poor sleep patterns and excessive frequency or uncontrolled patterns of urination. Similarly, deficiencies of other minerals, or imbalances in the levels of those minerals, can produce many other problems in the body.

That's why it's important to detoxify and clean the body through fasting and through using pure, distilled water as well as healthy, organically-grown vegetables and fruits and their juices. At the same time, it's also important to provide the body with adequate sources of new minerals. This can be accomplished by eating a wide variety of organic garden salads and vegetables. Also include kelp granules – great sprinkled over foods, salads, etc. and try other sea vegetables. These help produce healthy mother's milk for infants. Give the healthier Rice Dream, nut (almond, etc.) or soy milks to children and adults who are affected (mucus, colds, asthma, etc.) by milk products. We don't endorse using dairy products.

But despite dietary sources such as these, many adults and children in so-called civilized cultures will be found to have low levels of essential minerals in their bodies. These deficiencies are caused by coffee, tea, carbonated beverages, colas and long-term bad diets (too much sugar, refined flours, salt, additives, etc.)

In addition, the body's organ systems can be thrown out of balance by continuing stress and toxins in our air and water, and disease-produced injuries and by prenatal deficiencies in the mother's diet or lifestyle. As a result people may need to take a natural mineral supplement such as the chelated multiple mineral preparations and also a multiple vitamin supplement.

Supplements are good insurance to insure that you are getting enough minerals, vitamins and nutrients to maintain your health.

Ask Yourself These Vital Health Questions:

- How can I stop chemicals and inorganic minerals from hardening and turning my brain and body into stone?

- How can I stop my body's joints and back from becoming painful, stiff and cemented?

- How can I help stop the formation of gallstones, kidney stones and bladder stones?

- How can I protect my arteries, veins and capillaries from the unnatural, hardening of arteriosclerosis?

- How can I prolong my youthfulness?

- How can I prevent sickness and premature ageing?

To find the answer to these questions and more details on why I say "Drink pure distilled water," read the Bragg book *Water – The Shocking Truth That Can Save Your Life!*

164

Don't injure your system by over-feeding it.
Over-eating will kill you long before your time.

Nothing transforms anyone as much as changing
from a negative to a positive attitude.

Fasting and prayer seemed to strengthen Jesus, for when His time of temptation and fasting was ended, He manifested a new power and poise. Jesus returned in the power of the Spirit into Galilee. – Luke 4:14

I humbled my soul with fasting. – Psalm 69:10

Avoid all self-drugging – such as aspirin and similar drugs, pain killers, sleeping pills, tranquilizers, antihistamines, milk of magnesia, laxatives, strong cathartics and fizzing bromides. You are not qualified to prescribe drugs for yourself (results can be serious). The best solution is to correct the health problems causing pain, constipation, etc. – Patricia Bragg

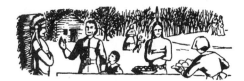

Chapter 22

Doctor Good Natural Food

Your body is the most gloriously accurate instrument in this universe. Given the correct fuel, pure air, exercise, sunshine and internal cleansing by fasting, your body will function perfectly and last almost indefinitely.

A healthy body is an efficient chemical factory. Given the correct raw materials, it should be capable (except for accidents) of developing strong tissues and good resistance against most bacteria, viruses and other environmental factors.

It is the only fine machine I know of that contains its own repair shop. It'll work wonders if you give it the proper tools! It is constantly working for you. Its cells are being destroyed and renewed every second. Biologically, it has no age limit. In fact, there is no biological reason for man to grow old at all. The body has the seed of eternal life. Man does not die. He commits slow suicide with his unhealthy habits of living.

165

Scientists tell us that almost every cell in our body is renewed every 11 months. Then why should anyone speak of being old? Don't you believe the moth-eaten fallacy that man, as he gets older, must face decrepitude, decay, senility and death! If people knew what to eat and only ate what they should, Old Father Time would shoulder his scythe and walk off in the other direction!

Most people are suffering from mineral and vitamin deficiencies. Research shows that millions are victims of malnutrition. The body's millions of red blood cells are constantly dying and being replaced; some are being renewed every second. They can't be rejuvenated properly without the right substances and these must come from healthy, natural foods.

The first wealth is health. – Emerson

Healthy Foods Build & Maintain Your Body!

The person you are today, tomorrow, next week, next month and 10 years from now depends on what you eat! You are the sum total of the food you consume. How you look, feel and carry your years all depends on what you eat! Every part of your body is made from food - the hair on your head, your eyes, teeth, bones, blood and flesh. Even your expression is formed from what you eat, because the healthy man is a well-fed, happy man. We often jokingly say, "What are we going to feed our faces?" when it is plain that we mean our entire bodies (including our faces) are ready for nourishment.

We can begin anywhere in the body, but it's best starting with the skeleton which supports all other tissues. Superficially, our bones are largely minerals – mostly calcium and phosphate. One might suppose that once the skeleton is formed, nutrition of the bone stops. This is far from true! Using "isotopic tracers" biochemists have found that, even in an adult body, minerals are constantly leaving and entering the bones. This means that bones are alive and are dynamic rather than static. Bones contain living cells which require not only minerals for building bone, but all the other food nutrients that living cells need to remain healthy.

An emergency need for these cells arises when a bone is broken. If these cells had ceased to live and function when the adult skeleton became formed, a broken bone would remain broken for the rest of one's life. When a bone is broken, nourishment of these cells is crucially important. They not only need the minerals required for repairing the damage, but the cells themselves need to "eat" and keep healthy. These bone cells, like all other cells, can be nourished at various levels of efficiency. This is related to the fact that bones sometimes knit slowly and sometimes rapidly. The rate of healing can be slowed dramatically by poor nutrition of the cells, or it can be stepped up by improving the cell's nutrition.

When recovering from accidents, fractures, etc. take extra mineral and vitamin supplements to help your body heal faster.

The Whole Body Needs Healthy Foods

Good physicians who treat fracture cases, especially doctors who are nutrition and health-minded make sure that every possible measure is taken to promote the finest nutrition possible to mend and build new bone cells.

The cells in our skin, including the hair-building cells, need continual healthy nourishment. This becomes more evident and compelling when we remember that skin is constantly being shed and replaced, and that hair grows continuously – day and night, year after year.

Those who handle farm animals, pets or racing animals know that skin and hair sleekness is an important index of health and well being. If an animal's hair or fur is well-nourished and healthy, it's an indication the cells of its body are at least fairly well nourished. Laboratory experiments with mammals and fowl show that many entirely different nutritional deficiencies will cause the skin, hair, or feathers, to become unhealthy. Doctors recognize the appearance of healthy skin and are often able to judge a patient's condition on this basis. Several gross vitamin deficiencies in humans become obvious by their unhealthy skin.

That national epidemic, constipation, is often a manifestation of bad nutrition of the intestinal tissues. There are many involuntary "smooth" muscles which, when stimulated, cause stomach and intestinal movements. These wavelike motions keep the partially digested food moving along until the final residue reaches the large bowel and is soon eliminated. All these smooth muscles are made up of living cells which must be well nourished if the whole process is to proceed with efficiency. In order to prevent constipation in the intestinal tract, irritating substances (powerful laxatives) are often used. These stimulate and "drive" the muscle cells, sometimes mercilessly, when usually all that the muscle cells need to function efficiently is some fiber and ample water, coupled with good nutritional habits.

Man does not die; he commits suicide with living an unhealthy lifestyle.
– Paul C. Bragg

The Body is a Mass of Living Cells

The system of arteries, veins and capillaries which carries blood and nourishment to all parts of the body are not inert pipes; their walls contain indispensable living cells which must be nourished satisfactorily in order to remain alive and well. They do not always stay well, as in the case of so-called hardening of the arteries that results from an unhealthy "corroded" condition which can be aggravated by improper nutrition.

The center of the circulatory system, the heart, is very much alive and its continual nourishment is crucially important. The heart is a powerful muscle which utilizes a tremendous amount of energy. Its cells need to be "fed" a highly nutritious "natural diet" day in and day out because it pumps blood all over the body. If an artery supplying blood to the heart becomes unhealthy and corroded, it is more likely to be stopped up by a small blood clot. In that case, the heart muscle cells which depend on the artery for sustenance are starved.

168

If the starvation, particularly for oxygen, is extensive and lasts even a fraction of a minute, the victim may die of a coronary heart attack. In this case, the quality of the blood may be satisfactory, but it cannot get through to the heart muscle cells, and thus cannot carry its nutrients to them. The heart cells die and this causes all the cells in the body to die. This is another example in which failure of cells to get what they need in one area can cause severe damage elsewhere in the body.

There are various special organs in the body that have extraordinary and distinctive nutritional requirements. All the important hormone-producing glands in the body (the thyroid gland, the pituitary, the adrenals, the sex glands, the insulin producing cells in the pancreas, the parathyroids) are made up of living cells. Like all other living cells, they need continuous and complex nourishment to keep the organs and body healthy.

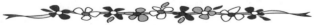

The greatest tragedy that comes to man is emotional depression, the dulling of the intellect and the loss of initiative that comes from nutritive failure. – Dr. James McLester, *Former A.M.A. President*

Iodine from Kelp is Important

One of these hormones is particularly interesting because it contains a specific chemical element – iodine. The cells that produce the thyroid hormone are among the most differentiated cells in the body . . . they absolutely need iodine if they are to perform their unique function. In certain parts of the world, such as the Great Lakes region, the Pacific Northwest and Switzerland, iodine is at a low level in soil and vegetation. As a result, many have thyroid glands that are relatively starved for iodine. They become diseased and highly swollen, resulting in the condition known as endemic goiter. They simply cannot do the job of producing the required hormone adequately unless they are furnished with enough iodine to create it. When sufficient iodine is furnished through supplements from sea vegetation (kelp, seaweed, Irish moss, etc.), the enlarged thyroid gland shrinks to normal size and the diseased condition disappears. Example: by limiting the different degrees of iodine given a mammal, it's possible to produce any condition between severe goiter and normal functioning.

The Effect of Good Food on the Brain

At first glance, no connection between food and thinking is apparent. Yet I assure you that, just as surely as food affects the different parts of the body, it also affects our thinking. Our thoughts are influenced directly by what we have eaten; especially what we eat habitually.

The brain is given credit for the processes of thought, though some profess to doubt this and maintain that thought originates outside of us, in the ethereal universe. But wherever it originates, the processes are certainly governed by some parts of the body. The brain occupies the most strategic position in the body for direction of thoughts and impulses. It is the logical seat for emotions, motivating impulses and conscious thinking.

The brain is the great reflex center, from which radiate all the nerves that control motion and sensation. Just as the brain depends on the blood for fresh oxygen, surely it must be affected by what we eat . . . for what we eat determines the sort of blood we have.

Alcohol, Toxins and Drugs Are Killers!

A brain nourished by blood full of toxic poisons isn't able to function at its greatest efficiency. Toxins can so befuddle the brain that clear thinking is impossible. Life-threatening comatose states can result from unusually deep types of intoxication, as in alcohol and drug overdoses.

To have a crystal clear, alert and sharp brain you must keep the toxic poisons in your blood at the lowest level possible. You must eat a diet that will supply all your brain cells with proper nourishment. Keeping toxic poisons at the lowest levels calls for regular fasting and a diet that supplies all the nutrients the brain needs.

Refined, Processed Foods, High in Fat, Salt & Sugar, Produce Learning Disabled Children

To demonstrate the effect that toxic poisons and malnutrition have on children, I have talked to many educators across America. They have thousands of children between the ages of 6 and 17 that are having difficulty being educated. Their brains are sick and slow from toxic poisons and malnutrition because of the standard American refined diet. These children have been fed on breakfast, lunch and dinner foods that have had all the nutrients refined out of them, then toxic preservatives added. Although the schools are blamed for turning out uneducated students, often this isn't the fault of the teacher. The blame lies on the parents for their children's unhealthy lifestyle!

Parents are often misled by TV, radio, magazine and newspaper advertising. These tell the parents to give the children processed foods which are largely composed of refined starch, sugar and fat. These "empty calorie" foods quickly satisfy a child's appetite, but contain practically no healthy nutrients.

Fasting regularly gives your organs a rest and helps reverse the ageing process for a longer and healthier life.
– James Balch, M.D. *Prescriptions for Nutritional Healing*

One fourth of what we eat keeps us, and the other three fourths we keep at the peril of our lives. – Abernethy

Worthless Enriched Breads & Cereals
Are Fed to American Children

They are told to give the children "Blunder bread" and "Ghost toasties" that have been "enriched." This is virtually an admission that essential food values have been extracted in the processing, and that the product needs to be "enriched." Mothers feed their children hot dogs, luncheon meats, refined, bleached breads that are all loaded with chemical additives! Children of today all drink sugared cola drinks. They are filled with "empty calories" which may give a short surge of quick energy, but they contain no basic health nutrients such as vitamins and minerals.

They eat commercial ice cream which is high in sugar and filled with toxic additives and commercial fillers. They eat candy bars, cookies, donuts, cakes and pastries. These foods could be called "deprived" foods. They satisfy a child by making him feel well-fed when he is truly being partly starved by spoiling his appetite for better, more nourishing healthy foods.

171

How in heaven's name can you feed a child's brain on such "junk foods" as potato chips or french fries with salt and gobs of catsup smeared over them? It's little wonder our nation's test scores are so low and still falling.

Most Young American Men Are Unfit

Is it any wonder that 58% of all the young men who enter the military service are physically unfit? The United States Army Planning Officer, stated, "Even though standards have not been raised, there is a worsening condition of the American youth. The percentages of failures due to their inability to meet minimum service requirements has been alarming."

The American Journal of Clinical Nutrition, flatly states that: "Nutrition is the most important single factor affecting health. This is true at age 1 or 101. But too often, this fact is overlooked in the development of new health programs. Nutrition is a specific factor in the prevention and control of many chronic diseases."

Medical Science notes that: "One of every 14 boys and 1 of every 17 girls under the age of 20 are hospitalized in a year and their hospital costs are high, according to the experience of one insurance company."

An editorial in the *London Times* said, "The food industry . . . is in for a turbulent time and had better take steps at once to remedy its shameful neglect of basic research in nutrition."

In *World Medical Journal,* Dr. G. Burch, Professor of Medicine at Tulane University, New Orleans, Louisiana, states, "Even in the young age group, the incidence of neoplastic diseases such as leukemia (cancer of the blood) is increasing. The collagen diseases such as acute arthritis are also becoming common among youth."

Boys made a sad showing in physical examinations while the nutritional status of girls – the mothers of tomorrow – is even more serious. Most nutritionists, doctors and teachers agree that basically two factors are to blame: dietary ignorance and the lack of parental direction. One of the immediate consequences is the inability to resist infectious disease. Childbirth complications are another result of poor nutrition. A woman whose nutrition is not adequate for her own body cannot expect to produce a healthy baby.

America leads the world in the highest standard of living, the largest supplies of food and highest health care costs. These factors should make it the healthiest nation in the world, not one of the sickest! Yet, America has the gloomiest health forecast and leads the world in degenerative diseases. Why? Maybe because Americans consume more processed, chemicalized, toxic foods than any other nation.

Three Needed Health Habits

There are 3 habits which, with but one condition added, will give you every thing in the world worth having, beyond which the imagination of man cannot conjure forth a single additional improvement! These habits are:
• **The Work Habit** • **The Health Habit** • **The Study Habit**
If you have these habits, and also have the love of someone who has these same habits, you are both in paradise now and here. – Elbert Hubbard

American Adults Are in a Sad Physical and Mental Condition

If you think school age children are befuddled in their thinking, consider the adult population. If you think the young population is half sick or completely ill, our adult population is even worse! I have noted that 58% of our youth between 18 and 25 would be unfit for military service. If we examined our adult population aged from 25 to 75, what a group of physical and mental wrecks we would find!

If a group of 15 adults are gathered together in a room for a social evening and the conversation turns to health and disease, you can be sure that 99% of these people have some chronic ailment eating away at one or more of their vital organs. It seems that everyone has something wrong with them! They talk of the shots they are taking, the operations they have had or are going to have, the pills they are taking and the misery they are suffering. They calmly admit to each other that they are seeing a therapist, as if it were natural to be in a confused condition!

173

The longer the adult person lives on the standard civilized diet, the worse he gets mentally and physically. This is proven by the many convalescent and nursing homes in America. These places are packed with prematurely old adults, many who are senile, feeble, forgetful humans. I ask you, "Is this the way that God and Mother Nature intended us to end our days on earth?" If you are going to eat a diet deficient in the essential nutrients and let your body become loaded with toxic poisons, the answer is, "Yes!" Just because we live a limited number of years, there is absolutely no need for us to break down mentally or physically.

Since the mind is supported by purely physical processes, it is not hard to see the connection between foods and thinking. Our physical functions depend so completely on what we eat that we cannot disassociate our state of mind from the quality of our foods.

The freedom and ease you experience during fasting enables you to discover new undreamed of depths to the meanings of life.
– Herbert Shelton

Mental, Physical and Spiritual Rewards

During fasts, when the body nears a purified state, the mind is on such a high level that the subconscious mind becomes very active and sharp. One can almost seem to experience the supernatural. Some of the greatest mental feats have been performed during a fast. Also higher mental efficiency has been noted for long periods following the fast. Because fasting clears the system of most toxic debris, the brain is nourished by a purer blood stream and reaches amazing heights of efficiency.

America has achieved miracles in inventions and science; but how much more might we have achieved if we had known the simple facts of fasting and proper nutrition as a foundation for thinking more efficiently?

The ancient Greek philosophers placed proper diet first in training their students. Their rigid use of foods shows clearly it's importance in their philosophy. Socrates, Epicurus, Plato and many others placed great emphasis on fasting and food and its relation to the mind as a background for philosophical study. They practiced what they preached – they fasted regularly.

174

The philosophy of these sages is respected today as thinking on a very high plane. It's been said that the sayings of these men contained wisdom so far advanced that it appeared divinely inspired! I believe this.

Out of a toxic body come foul, evil thoughts and, conversely, a clean, purified body emits clean thoughts. The responsibility for clear thinking arises from the quality of eating along with living a healthy lifestyle.

As the body becomes cleared of toxic debris, we begin to think on a higher plane. **"As a man thinketh in his heart, so is he,"** is more than a trite saying. When the body is cleared of waste material, the mind soars to heights not formerly glimpsed by toxin-filled minds. New worlds open to the cleansed, reborn body and mind.

Healthy, healing dietary fibers are fresh vegetables, fresh fruits, salads and whole grains and their products. These health builders help to normalize blood pressure, cholesterol and promote healthy elimination.

Healthy Eating is a Science!

Most of the worthwhile things in life are those things that have helped others. The greatest accomplishments for ages have been achieved by those who placed accomplishment before idle pleasure! You will never find gluttons among those great minds who eat a devitalized, processed or dead food diet.

Eating should be a science and of first importance to everyone. Eating is such a fundamental thing. We depend on food for efficiency, health, happiness and longevity. Good nutrition should be a basic rule of every person's early training . . . to eat for health.

It's never too late to start eating natural foods and living The Bragg Healthy Lifestyle. The minute you begin a natural diet, your body, mind and spirit will start to improve! In 11 short months you can build a whole, new, wonderful, youthful feeling body by fasting to clean out the half-dead cells and using natural foods to build new, youthful cells. This is the great secret of life.

You will become the Master Builder of a brand new body, free from miseries! You will develop a sharp and alert brain. Your spirit – your soul, will soar to greater heights! There is no greater treasure than living on the highest planes of the physical, mental and the spiritual existence. Doctor Good Natural Food will be your guide to achieve the Higher Life. Trust in Him, for He wants you to have a perfect healthy life while you're on earth.

175

CREATIVE MEDICINE

It is no over-simplification to say that our health comes from the soil. No matter how many physicians and health professionals we train, and how much curative or preventative medicine they may practice, we cannot attain optimum health until our attention is focused on preventive medicine, and thereby learn to keep and even improve our health. To build and maintain healthy soil is the real fundamental service. Creative medicine must be founded on growing healthy organic foods. Thus alone can we create real health for our people – only through creating a sound, healthy and prosperous organic-minded agriculture.

– Dr. Jonathan Foreman, *The Land*

It is never too late to be what you might have been. – George Elliot

Healthy Fiber for Super Health

- EAT BERRIES, surprisingly good sources of fiber.
- KEEP BEANS HANDY, probably the best fiber sources. Cook dried beans and freeze in portions. Use canned beans for faster meals.
- INSTEAD OF ICEBERG LETTUCE, choose deep green lettuces, romaine, bib, butter, etc., spinach or cabbage for variety salads.
- LOOK FOR "100% WHOLE WHEAT" or whole grain breads. A dark color isn't proof; check labels, compare fibers, grains, etc.
- WHOLE GRAIN CEREALS. Hot, also cold granolas with sliced fruit.
- GO FOR BROWN RICE. It's better for you and so delicious.
- EAT THE SKINS of potatoes and other fruits and vegetables.
- LOOK FOR CRACKERS with at least 2 grams of fiber per ounce.
- SERVE HUMMUS, made from chickpeas, instead of sour-cream dips.
- USE WHOLE WHEAT FLOUR for baking breads, muffins, pastries, pancakes, waffles and for variety try other whole grain flours.
- DON'T UNDERESTIMATE CORN, including popcorn, corn tortillas.
- ADD OAT BRAN, WHEAT BRAN AND WHEATGERM to baked goods, cookies, etc.; whole grain cereals, casseroles, loafs, etc.

- SNACK ON SUN-DRIED FRUIT, such as apricots, dates, prunes, raisins, etc., which are concentrated sources of nutrients and fiber.
- INSTEAD OF DRINKING JUICE, eat the fruit: orange, grapefruit, etc.; and vegetables: tomato, carrot, etc. – UC Berkeley Wellness Letter

Most Common Food Allergies

- *CEREALS: Buckwheat, Corn, Oats, Rye, Wheat*
- *MILK: Butter, Cheese, Cottage Cheese, Ice Cream, Milk, etc.*
- *EGGS: Cakes, Custards, Dressings, Mayonnaise, Noodles*
- *FISH: Shellfish, Crabs, Lobster, Shrimp, Shadroe*
- *MEATS: Bacon, Chicken, Pork, Sausage, Veal*
- *FRUITS: Citrus Fruits, Melons, Strawberries*
- *VEGETABLES: Brussels Sprouts, Cauliflower, Celery, Eggplant, Legumes, Onions, Potatoes, Spinach, Tomatoes*
- *NUTS: Peanuts, Pecans, Walnuts*
- *MISCELLANEOUS: Chocolate, China Tea, Cocoa, Coffee, Palm and Cottonseed Oils, MSG, Salt, Spices*

Nature's Wonder Working Phytochemicals Help Prevent Cancer

Make sure to get your daily dose of these naturally occurring, cancer fighting biological substances, that are abundant in onions, garlic, beans, legumes, soybeans, cabbage, cauliflower, broccoli, citrus fruits, etc. The winner is tomatoes, which alone contain about 10,000 different phytochemicals!

Chapter 23

Doctor Fasting

Fasting is accepted and recognized as being the oldest form of therapy. It is mentioned 74 times in the Bible. It is the universal therapy even used by sick animals in the wilds the world over. As we study the ancient healers of the world, we find that fasting heads the list for helping Mother Nature heal the sick and the wounded.

There is a misconception about fasting that must be clarified. It must be definitely and positively stated that fasting is not a cure for any disease or ailment. The purpose of a fast is to allow the body's Vital Force full range and scope to fulfill its own self-healing, self-repairing and self-rejuvenating functions to the best advantage. Healing is an internal biological function. Fasting gives the body a physiological rest and permits the body to become 100% efficient in healing itself. Fasting under proper care or with workable knowledge is probably the fastest way and the safest means of regaining health ever conceived by the human mind!

177

Even if I have to repeat myself, I want to make it clear and positive that fasting does not cure anything. Fasting puts the body in a condition where all the Vital Force of the body is used to flush out the causes of body miseries. Fasting helps the body help itself. We who have made a life study of the Science of Fasting and conducted and supervised thousands of fasts know the miracles that the body itself can perform during the period of complete abstinence from food. It gives the overworked and overburdened internal organs rest and time for rehabilitation. It enhances the internal power and vitality of the body to flush out toxic poisons and wastes that have been stored in the body for years. It raises the

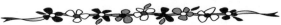

On a fast day . . . you shall read the words of the Lord. – Jeremiah 36:6

Vital Force to its highest point of efficiency. Thus, it promotes the elimination of inorganic chemical accumulations and other pollutions that cannot be flushed from the body by any other means.

The prophets of old fasted for spiritual enlightenment and a closer contact with the Godhead (Divine Force). We know that fasting sharpens and hones the mental faculties to a keen edge. Fasting improves the organs of mastication, digestion, assimilation and elimination of food. The mighty liver – which is known as the chemical laboratory of the human body and is typically the most abused organ – at last has a chance during the fast to rehabilitate and gain more Vital Force. Thus, after a fast, the liver functions more efficiently. In particular, all the sensory powers possessed by human beings are exhilarated and raised to a much higher efficiency level than normal during and after a fast.

No process of therapy ever fulfilled so many indications for restoration of vigorous health as does fasting. It is Mother Nature's very own prime process and her first requirement in nearly all cases. After a fast the circulation is better, food can be assimilated better, while endurance, stamina and strength are increased. After a fast the mind becomes more receptive to logic and a sensible, natural way of living.

After the fast the mind becomes so powerful that it can take full control of the body. It becomes the complete master and, if a person does not go back to his old habits, he can maintain this mastery of the body for the rest of his life. Fasting instills personal confidence. Fasting gives a person a positive mental attitude. Fasting promotes tranquility of mind and a glow of well-being that no other therapy can offer. Fasting renovates, revives and purifies every one of the millions of cells that make up the body. Fasting is the Royal Road to Internal Purity!

Actress Cloris Leachman is an ardent health follower who sparkles with health. She hates smoking, coffee, alcohol, sugar and meat. One of her solutions to health problems is to fast. "Fasting is simply wonderful. I can do practically anything. It is a miracle cure. It cured my asthma."

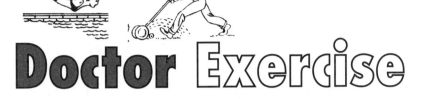

Chapter 24

Doctor Exercise

Doctor Exercise makes this statement, "To rest is to rust!" And rust means decay and destruction. In other words, the good doctor tells us that activity is life and stagnation is death. The good doctor further informs us that if we do not use our muscles, we lose them! In order to keep muscles firm, strong, vigorous and youthful, they must be continually used. Activity is the law of life! Action is the law of well-being. Every vital organ of the body has its specialized work, and its performance depends on its development and strength.

When we use the body, we build endurance, strength and vigor. When we become lazy and do not use our muscles, we bring on decay and death. Daily exercise quickens and equalizes the circulation of the blood, but in laziness, the blood does not circulate freely and the changes in it that are so vital to life and health do not take place. We have poor muscle tone and the muscles become flabby and unable to perform vigorous activity.

People who do not exercise often have poor skin tone. Exercise brings on healthy perspiration in the 96 million pores of our body. The skin is the largest eliminative organ in the entire body. If someone would shellac or gild your body and thus clog the pores, you would die within a few minutes. With exercise, you bring on healthy perspiration. Impurities and toxins are expelled when you exercise and perspire freely – you are allowing the skin to perform its natural function of eliminating poisons. If you don't exercise daily to the point of perspiring, the work that the pores are not doing throws a double burden on the other eliminative organs and then you get into health problems.

Kindness should be a frame of mind in which we are alert to every chance to do, to give, to share and to cheer.

179

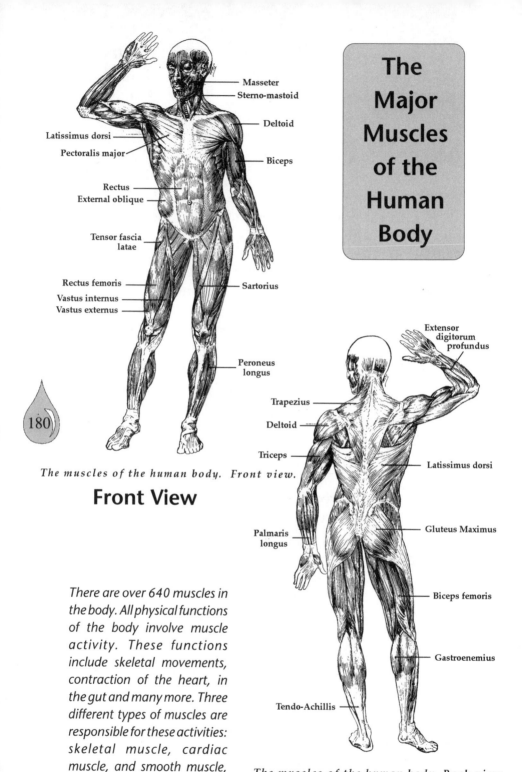

The Major Muscles of the Human Body

Masseter
Sterno-mastoid
Deltoid
Latissimus dorsi
Pectoralis major
Biceps
Rectus
External oblique
Tensor fascia latae
Rectus femoris
Vastus internus
Vastus externus
Sartorius
Peroneus longus

180

The muscles of the human body. Front view.

Front View

Extensor digitorum profundus
Trapezius
Deltoid
Triceps
Latissimus dorsi
Palmaris longus
Gluteus Maximus
Biceps femoris
Gastroenemius
Tendo-Achillis

The muscles of the human body. Back view.

Back View

There are over 640 muscles in the body. All physical functions of the body involve muscle activity. These functions include skeletal movements, contraction of the heart, in the gut and many more. Three different types of muscles are responsible for these activities: skeletal muscle, cardiac muscle, and smooth muscle, all of which have some characteristics in common.

Exercise Normalizes Blood Pressure

Exercise helps to normalize blood pressure and create a healthy pulse. Exercise is an anticoagulant, meaning that it keeps the blood from clotting (called a "thrombus" which often brings on a heart attack).

Every creature seeking to eliminate internal waste does so by means of muscular action. Inside your intestines there are 3 muscular layers which undergo a rhythmic, wavelike action called peristalsis. A serious condition results if you allow the internal and external muscles, through inactivity, to become flabby and fat instead of muscular. The muscles lose their tone and power to contract, resulting in intestinal clogging. The abdominal muscles play an important role in the evacuation effort. What happens when the internal and external muscles become flabby, soft, sick and infiltrated with fat? They refuse to work and we pile up intestinal waste that should have been eliminated. This brings about autointoxication, or the building of large amounts of toxic poison. Again, inactivity is the avoidable cause of many diseases.

Fasting and diet are 2 allies in your struggle for long lasting youth, health and symmetry. When it comes to fighting fat, diet and fasting come first. But when it comes to keeping fit, it is exercise that matters most! However, they all help each other, for by exercising regularly you may be more generous in your diet and, up to a certain point, your extra food will make for increased vitality. The human machine should work at the highest pitch of efficiency. As with all machines, it improves with intelligent use. Nothing betrays its weak spots like inactivity and rust.

Walking for Health, Fitness and Life

I believe in all of the many forms of exercise, but without hesitation I will tell you that walking is the best all-around exercise. Of all forms of exercise, walking is the one that brings most of the body into action.

Don't injure your system by over-feeding it.
Over-eating will kill you long before your time.

Walking – The King of Exercise

As you walk, grasp yourself in the small of the back and feel how your entire frame responds to every stride. Notice how almost all of your muscles are functioning rhythmically. No other exercise gives us the same body harmony of movement and improved circulation. Brisk walking is the best exercise for almost everyone.

Your walking should never be done consciously. No "heel and toe" business. No getting there in a certain time. Let it be fun and natural. Of course, you will carry yourself well. Walk naturally with your head high and chest up. You will feel physically elated, so you will carry yourself proudly, straight, erect and with arms swinging.

Vow to become a wonderful walker and make the daily walk a fixed item in your health program all the year around, in all kinds of weather. Go at your own stride with your spirit free. If the outer world of nature fails to interest you, turn to the inner world of the mind. As you walk, your body ceases to matter and you become as near poet and philosopher as you will ever be. Each to his own taste, but to my mind this is better than golf! Life has so much to teach us that it is a pity to waste big chunks of time trying to get a ball into a hole in a stroke less than the other fellow. However the end is the same, the healthy functioning of muscles and quickened blood circulation with a sense of harmony and happiness.

Gardening is another marvelous form of exercise. It will give you enough exercise in the open to help keep you in good physical condition. But gardening may not prevent weight gain if there is too little movement and because you are bent over more instead of being erect. For this reason, I prefer walking. But perhaps some of both is best for you. Satisfy your conscience by applying your energy productively in your health garden, then take the kink out of your back with a healthy walk. In my personal life, I combine a system of calisthenics with brisk walking and running to stay in good shape.

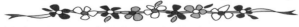

Fasting is Mother Nature and God's Miracle – it cleanses, renews & rejuvenates!

The Importance of Abdominal Exercises

I believe that the most important exercises are those that stimulate all of the muscles of the human trunk from the hips to the armpits. These are the binding muscles which hold all of the vital organs in place. When you develop your torso's muscles, you are also developing your internal muscles. As your back, waist, chest and abdomen increase in strength and elasticity, so will your lungs, liver, heart, stomach and kidneys gain in efficiency.

The widened arch of your ribs will give free play to your lungs. Your elastic diaphragm will allow your heart to pump more powerfully. Your rubber-like waist will, in its limber action, stimulate your kidneys and massage your liver. Your abdominal muscles will strengthen and support your stomach with controlled undulations. All of this hard, clean development of your torso will stimulate the sound walls of your house and fortify the interior to resist the ravages of time. Trunk exercise acts like a massage of the vital organs. For that reason alone, it has a positive influence over the whole organism that cannot be underestimated.

183

The more you fast, the more poison you clean from your body. As your body increases in internal cleanliness, your muscles have more tone and vitality. You will find after a fast that the old sluggish, lazy feeling is gone and, in its place, there will be a desire for more action and more physical activity. You bubble with energy.

Should You Exercise While Fasting?

This is a question which only the faster can answer. If there is no inclination for physical activity during a fast, then you should not exercise. The fast is giving you a physiological rest and – unless you have a tremendous, overwhelming urge for physical activity – you should rest as much as possible. Your body is using all of its Vital Force for internal purification. But if you should feel, during a 7 to 10 day fast, that you need some stretching or walking, by all means respond to the urge. It is between fasts and in your daily program of living that you should spend a portion of every day of your life pursuing outdoor exercises. Between fasts, you must substitute vigorous circulation for sluggish circulation, for it's the main cause of much discomfort, pain and misery in the body.

When people don't exercise, their ankles and legs often swell because there is not enough blood circulation to remove the waste from the cells and carry it back to the organs of elimination. There should be no excuse for not exercising because, regardless of your physical condition, it's vitally important that exercise be a part of your life. Daily exercise prevents sickness and premature ageing. It builds a fund of endurance and resistance. It helps build a strong heart and a rich bloodstream, giving proper balance of white and red corpuscles to attack and overcome any harmful germs that may invade the body.

Exercise helps to maintain a serene and tranquil mind. A 5 mile walk in the fresh air will help to neutralize any unhealthy emotional upset. Exercise increases confidence, for there is no better way to supreme confidence than the satisfying knowledge of improved mental and physical abilities. Exercise gives you a positive attitude. It cultivates willpower and it gives absolute mastery of your physical, mental and spiritual self which promotes personal efficiency.

Exercise is the greatest health tonic one can give oneself! You will attain the feeling of radiant, glorious living by following your fasting program and exercise regime. You will feel better and look better! Satisfying the body's craving for physical activity produces the miraculous feeling of agelessness.

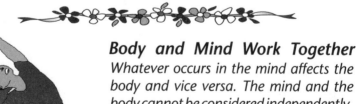

Body and Mind Work Together
Whatever occurs in the mind affects the body and vice versa. The mind and the body cannot be considered independently. When the two are out of sync, both emotional and physical stress can erupt.
– Hippocrates, The Father of Medicine

Iron Pumping Oldsters (86 to 96) Triple Their Muscle Strength in U.S. Study

WASHINGTON, In a 1990 landmark study – Ageing nursing home residents in Boston study "pumping iron"! Elderly weightlifters tripling and quadrupling their muscle strength? Is it possible? Most people would doubt it! But government experts on ageing answered those questions with a resounding "yes" thanks to the results of this amazing landmark study!

They turned a group of frail Boston nursing home residents, aged 86 to 96, into weightlifters to demonstrate that it's never too late to reverse age-related declines in muscle strength. The group participated in a regimen of high-intensity weight-training in a study conducted by the Agriculture Department's Human Nutrition Research Center on Ageing at Tufts University in Boston. "A high-intensity weight-training program is capable of inducing dramatic increases in muscle strength in frail men and women up to 96 years of age," reported Dr. Maria A. Fiatarone, who headed the study.

185

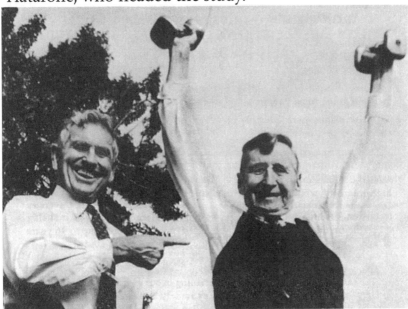

Paul C. Bragg and Friend, Roy White, 106 Years Young

Paul and Roy practiced progressive weight training 3 times a week to stay healthy and fit. Scientists have proven that weight training works miracles for all ages by maintaining more flexibility, energy and youthful stamina!

Amazing Body Strength Results in 8 Weeks

"The favorable response to strength training in our subjects was remarkable in light of their advanced ages, extremely sedentary habits, multiple chronic diseases, functional disabilities and nutritional inadequacies. The elderly weight-lifters increased their muscle strength by anywhere from three-fold to four-fold in as little as eight weeks." Fiatarone said that many were stronger at the end of the program than they had been in years!

Fiatarone and her associates emphasized the safety of such a closely supervised weight-lifting program, even among people in frail health. The average age of the 10 participants, for instance, was 90. Six had coronary heart disease; seven had arthritis; six had bone fractures resulting from osteoporosis; four had high blood pressure; and all had been physically inactive for years. Yet, no serious medical problems resulted from the weight-training program, only positive outcomes!

Study Shows Fitness Improves Wellness

A few of the patients did report minor muscle and joint aches, but 9 of the 10 completed the program. One man, aged 86, felt a pulling sensation at the site of a previous hernia incision and dropped out after 4 weeks.

The study participants, drawn from a 712 bed long-term care facility in Boston, worked out 3 times a week. They performed 3 sets of 8 repetitions with each leg on a weight-lifting machine. The weights were gradually increased from about 10 pounds initially to about 40 pounds at the end of the eight week program.

Fiatarone said the study carries some important implications to improve the wellness and fitness of older people, who represent a growing proportion of the U.S. population. A decline in muscle strength and size is one of the more predictable features of premature ageing.

Muscle strength in the average adult decreases by 30% to 50% during the course of life. Experts on ageing do not know whether the decrease is an unavoidable consequence of ageing or results mainly from sedentary lifestyle and other controllable factors.

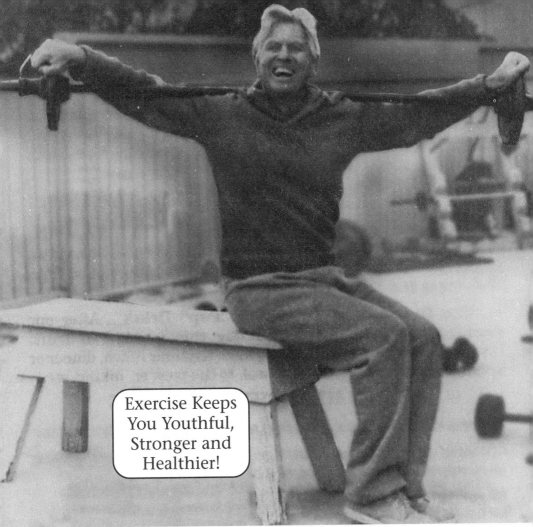

Exercise Keeps You Youthful, Stronger and Healthier!

Paul C. Bragg Lifts Weights 3 Times a Week

Muscle atrophy and weakness are not merely cosmetic problems in elderly people, especially the frail elderly. Researchers have linked muscle weakness with recurrent falls, a major cause of immobility and death in the American elderly population. This is results in millions of dollars yearly in staggering medical costs.

187

Previous studies have suggested that weight-training can be helpful in reversing age-related muscle weakness. But Fiatarone said physicians have been reluctant to recommend weightlifting for frail elderly with multiple health problems. This new government study might be changing their minds. Also, this study shows the great importance of keeping the 640 muscles as active and fit as possible to maintain general good health.

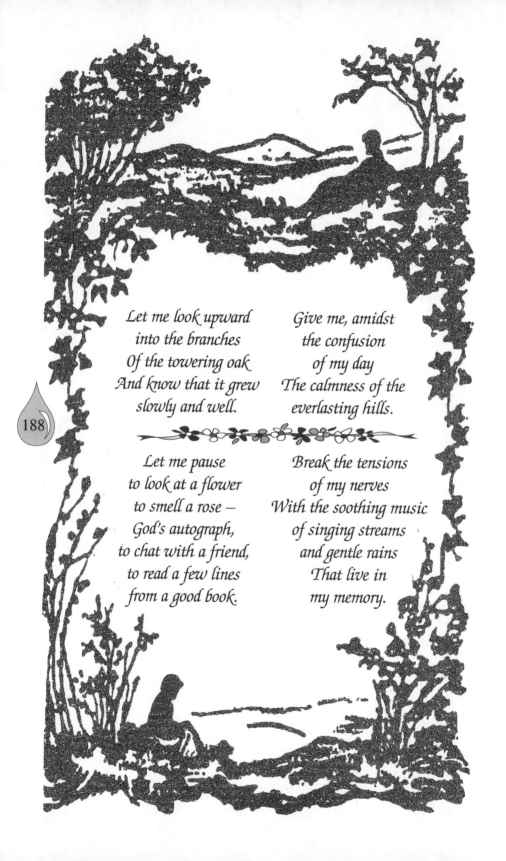

Let me look upward
into the branches
Of the towering oak
And know that it grew
slowly and well.

Give me, amidst
the confusion
of my day
The calmness of the
everlasting hills.

Let me pause
to look at a flower
to smell a rose —
God's autograph,
to chat with a friend,
to read a few lines
from a good book.

Break the tensions
of my nerves
With the soothing music
of singing streams
and gentle rains
That live in
my memory.

188

Chapter 25

Doctor Rest

Doctor Rest is another specialist who is always at your command to help you win Supreme Vitality. I believe the word "rest" is the most misunderstood word in the dictionary. Some people's idea of resting is to sit down and drink a cup of a strong stimulant such as alcohol, coffee, tea or soft drinks. This is particularly evident in the modern coffee break for employees. Rest means repose, freedom from activity, quiet and tranquility to me. It means peace of mind and spirit. It means to rest without anxiety or worry. It means to refresh oneself. Your rest should refresh your whole nervous system.

It does not mean sitting with one leg crossed over the other. When you sit with your legs crossed you are putting a tremendous burden on the main artery that supplies the feet with blood. You also cut off nerve energy. So if you sit with one leg crossed over the other you are not resting – you are giving the heart a tremendous load of work to do! Don't cross your legs when you sit down – keep both feet on the floor!

189

To properly rest and be still, it's also important to wear no restricting garments that might hinder your blood circulation. Are your shoes too tight? Your collar? Your hat? Your belt? Your undergarments?∗ Your stockings? If so, then you are not really resting when you sit still or lie down. The best rest is secured when you have loose or better yet very little clothing. Any clothes and shoes you are wearing should be comfortably loose and never binding.

Help me to know the magic of rest and relaxation and the restoring power of sleep.

∗Read *Dressed To Kill,* by Sydney Singer, on breast cancer & bra studies.

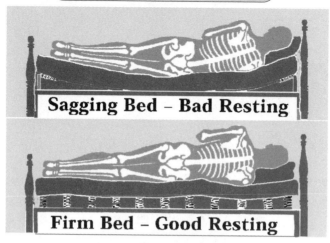

CHECK YOUR MATTRESS

Sagging Bed – Bad Resting

Firm Bed – Good Resting

Why Do We Rest?

190

You often hear people say "I must take a break." But when they sit down to rest, they nervously thump their fingers on a table or desk or they squirm and move restlessly. The art of resting must be acquired and concentrated upon. Among the best of the various ways you can rest is to lie down on a firm bed or couch unclothed or with as few loose clothes as possible. Another fine way to rest is take a sunbath because, if there is anything that will relax the muscles and nerves, it's the soothing gentle rays of the sun. You must learn to clear your mind of anxiety, worries and emotional problems. When muscles and nerves relax, the heart action slows – especially when you take slow, deep breaths. This will bring deep relaxation and total rest.

Another form of resting is a short nap. When taking this nap, you should command your muscles to become completely relaxed. Your mind controls your muscles and the nerves, so you must be in complete command of your body when you rest. The Master Teacher said to His Disciples, when they were worn and weary, "Come Ye and Rest a While." The Master did not lead them into the busy streets of Jerusalem where there was noise and clatter. He didn't even take them into the synagogue, but into the quiet of the wide open spaces, under the

The Lord gives strength to those who are weary. – Isaiah 40:29

blue sky. Here they could rebuild, relax and revive every organ of their exhausted bodies and revitalize, refresh, and invigorate their weary minds. Under the blue sky in the clean, fresh air is the greatest place to relax, rest and renew your Vital Force.

Sleep is the greatest revitalizer, but so few people get a long, peaceful and refreshing night's sleep. Most people habitually use stimulants: tobacco, drugs, coffee, tea, alcohol and cola drinks. All of these whip the tired nerves, so that people who use these stimulants can never have complete rest and relaxation because their nerves are always in an excited condition.

Rest Must Be Earned

Most people do not earn their rest. Rest is something that must be earned with physical and mental activity, because they go hand in hand. Many people have come to me seeking help, telling me what poor sleepers they are and how they roll and toss all night long. Today, millions of people regularly take some type of drug to induce sleep – but this is not true sleep. No one can get restful sleep from a drug! You may drug yourself into unconsciousness, but you cannot drug yourself into a restful, normal, healthy and satisfying sleep.

191

A body full of toxins is a constant irritant to the nerves. How is it possible to get a good night's rest with irritated nerves? In my many years of experience with fasting I found when people discard their stimulants when fasting, they become deep, restful sleepers. You will notice as you purify your body you will be able to relax more. You will be able to enjoy naps and enjoy the benefits of restful, night sleeps. Rest is important! The Bible tells us that God appointed one day of rest every week for man, an important factor in the maintenance of super health. Along with our busy days, we must add recreation to our activities. We have all heard the saying, "All work and no play makes Jack a dull boy."

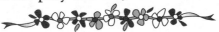

Honey whets the appetite, and so does wisdom! When you enjoy becoming wise, there is hope for you! – Proverbs 24:13-14

Life is To Be Enjoyed! Not Hectic & Rushed

Today we live in a mad, competitive world which is called "The Rat Race." It is dog-eat-dog, so we build up tremendous pressures, tensions, stresses and strains. I believe this is the reason why so many people turn to tobacco, drugs, coffee, alcohol and other stimulants. There is not only competition in the business world, but the desire to uphold status.

People are always trying to impress one another and create an image. Thus, a false image is created and it takes a tremendous amount of energy to portray a false image! Women told that gray hair makes them look old spend time and money being a slave to having their hair colored. They constantly try to keep up with the latest fashions. This all calls for energy. Often others push us beyond our limits and stress us out!

It's no wonder we have created 15 million chronic alcoholics and millions of drug addicts. Have we completely forgotten that life is to be lived, to be enjoyed? Leisurely living is something few people in our society enjoy. Life is rush and more rushing. Where are we rushing to? Where? In this hectic age – maybe the hospital or cemetery.

Plan, plot and follow through so your days have time for rest, recreation, exercise and a good night's sleep. You can't get a good night's sleep if you overload your stomach. Your body will have a good night's sleep if you have some vigorous, out-of-door exercise such as a brisk 2 mile walk, garden work, etc. It's vital to nourish your body with pure, natural foods and distilled water. Let it have plenty of fresh air and sunlight. Have a balanced program of exercise and repose. Let Mother Nature do the rest. Treat yourself as if you were a fine, purebred race horse and, as surely as it will win prizes, so will you! It's all too easy to sneer and laugh at the "back to Nature" people, but we who believe in Mother Nature will always have the last laugh.

Knowing these teachings will mean true life and good health for you.
– Proverbs 4:22

Mother Nature Knows What's Best!

One of the predominant suggestions of this book is a gradual return to Mother Nature and her natural way of living. In food, clothing, rest, sleep and a simplicity in living habits, try to reach a nearness to Mother Nature that makes you almost one with her. When you feel that the same pure forces that express themselves in a pine tree are expressing themselves in you, you have made a big stride toward a healthy ideal.

Begin to live as Mother Nature wants you to live. Seek to feel that she claims you and you are part of all glad, growing things. Put yourself into her hands and let her have her way with you. Leave to the young the smog-filled, air-polluted and microbe-infested cities. You will rekindle your own youth in the quiet beauty of hill and meadow. If you would grow young, begin by believing you can and that Mother Nature is eager to aid you. Better than any human or divine agency, she can run that ill-used machine of yours and, if it breaks down while in her hands, it is because its usefulness is really at an end. If you are a prisoner of the city, make it a point to get out to the country or the seashore where you can really find true rest, tranquillity and serenity.

193

In a brotherly way, I have tried to stress these points. First, you should demand of yourself a higher standard of health and happiness. You cannot receive higher health unless your body gets its rest periods to develop new vitality and energy. Second, you should regard your body as a machine under your care and control. Every machine must have rest periods. If not, you will build up too much friction. That is what we do in our lives. We build up too much nerve irritation. Third, with increasing years, you should draw closer and more intimately to Mother Nature. You should cease to look for thrills and over-stimulation; instead, seek a peaceful life. By living in simplicity and purity, you will be filled with more peace, joy and love.

A fool thinks he needs no advice, but a wise man listens to others.
– Proverbs 12:15

Nervous Tension can ruin your health in dozens of ways and diminish your productivity and even shorten your life span. – Dr. E. Jacobson, *You Must Relax*

Relax and Enjoy Your Life – It's No Crime

Let health, air, sun and complete rest work for you. With a serene clear eye and confidence, put yourself in Mother Nature's hands. Let her run your machine, heal your hurts and comfort you in sickness and adversity. Then, when you have lived a long life of usefulness and happiness, let her call you back home. Make Mother Nature your partner and – when you are resting, relaxing, and recreating new energy – she will always be there with her kind hand on your shoulder. So be a child of Mother Nature. Don't look for sophisticated thrills, but find your fun and diversion in relaxation and other pursuits that are simple, down to earth and one with Mother Nature. Your rewards will be many – including renewed health, a calmness of spirit and a new awareness of the perfect natural beauties that Mother Nature has bestowed upon us so generously.

194

In America we are prone to look down on the person who wants to relax or live a leisurely life, they are called lazy. It seems that we must be doing something constantly. We must be talking, listening to music, watching television, etc. We have to attend parties, movies, programs and athletic events of all kinds. We are constantly pushing and driving our bodies. No wonder so many people have emotional problems. The psychiatrists and the psychologists are all overworked. It's because we ourselves are overworked! Please don't be ashamed to relax to get off the hectic treadmill. It's not only fun to do nothing – it's healthful and necessary.

You have a natural, built-in tranquilizer located in the muscle cells which you should be using. Don't expect to take sedatives and still be skilled in relaxation. Barbiturates and true relaxation are not bedfellows! But I have known people who needed sedatives for at least 6 months and after fasting they were able to discard them.

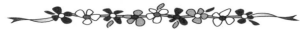

What sunshine is to flowers, smiles are to humanity. – Joseph Addison

Breathing deeply, fully and completely energizes the body, it calms the nerves, fills you with peace and helps keep you youthful. – Paul C. Bragg

Some Relaxation Techniques

To relax yourself to sleep, darken the room and turn off the TV or radio. Then lie flat on your back, hands down at sides without touching your body, to reduce sensory stimulation to a minimum. Let your hands rest, palms down, on the bed. Your legs should be extended with the feet approximately a foot apart. Your head may rest on a small pillow or directly on the bed, whichever is more comfortable. Permit your eyes to remain open at first, looking at an area, not at a point, directly in front of you – that is, on the opposite wall or ceiling, not up or down or to either side.

After the movements of your eyes have ceased, blinking movements of the lids may continue for a while. These won't interfere with the relaxation of the eye muscles. Thinking is always accompanied by eye movements. By relaxing your eyelids and eye muscles, you are slowing down your thought processes – and the end result of relaxation of the eyes and of other parts of the body is a natural, quiet and restorative sleep. If you have insomnia, reading just before going to sleep or reading to put yourself to sleep is not helpful because your eye muscles are probably already over-fatigued. Reading will tire them more, increasing the eye muscle tension and interfering with the process of relaxation which, uninterrupted, would inevitably lead to sleep.

195

Avoid Interruptions

Disregard all minor muscular discomforts while lying perfectly still and permit all of your muscles to relax without interruption. Don't tighten or move any muscles unless absolutely necessary. Movements of an arm or leg, or a change in your position, will interrupt the entire relaxation process and those muscles which have already attained a certain degree of relaxation must then begin the process all over again. Muscles that are tense may be uncomfortable, but if you move them you will only prolong their discomfort. Permit them to relax and the distress should disappear within 10 to 15 minutes.

Nothing in all creation is so like God as stillness. – Meister Eckhart

A relaxed muscle is a comfortable muscle and, if you are relaxing efficiently, you will feel comfortable. Discomfort in muscles is an indication that it is tense and that you are not permitting it to relax.

Insomnia Will Vanish

Those who are willing to devote 15 minutes a day in training themselves to relax can learn to break the insomnia habit, if they will faithfully follow The Bragg Healthy Lifestyle with the fasting program. Insomnia usually responds to relaxation techniques within 10 days. Then sweet, beautiful sleep will be yours every night. You will wake up in the glorious morning as bright and fresh as a healthy, newborn baby!

In the practice of relaxation, beginners have told me many times that they cannot possibly lie on their backs and go to sleep in that position. In observing the training of several hundred individuals, I have yet to prove the truth of that statement. If this is your belief, disregard it, for no matter how deeply entrenched this idea may be in your mind, you will be able to prove it is false.

"I always have to sleep on my right side." "I always sleep on my stomach." "I must curl up when I sleep." "I have to change my position frequently." "I cannot sleep at night if I have a nap in the daytime." "I must have my hand resting on my stomach." "I can go to sleep when I go to bed, but I wake up around 2 or 3 am and can't go back to sleep." "I sleep until 5 am, but then I am wide awake until I get up at 7 am and then am tired out by afternoon." Here's some common complaints we hear. (My wake up time is usually 5 am.)

Your fasting program is going to help you secure complete rest, relaxation and sound, sweet sleep. Toxins put pressure on your nerves and muscles. Fasting releases these pressures and allows your body to relax.

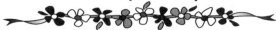

"Relieved of the work of digesting foods, fasting permits the body to rid itself of toxins while facilitating healing. Fasting regularly gives your organs a rest and helps reverse the ageing process for a longer and healthier life. Bragg books were my conversion to the healthy way."
– James Balch, M.D., *Prescription for Nutritional Healing*

Chapter 26

Doctor Good Posture

Why should emphasis be placed upon resisting the pull of gravity? This is very easy to explain. In the past, as long as your muscles were strong enough they held up your skeleton – with its many points and sections – in proper balance and free from strain or discomfort. Maybe now your muscles are losing the battle with gravity. Maybe you are prematurely older, heavier or inactivity has weakened your muscles just enough to cause you pain and an uncomfortable state of balance.

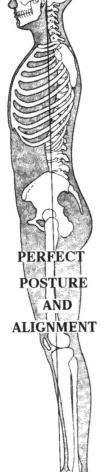

PERFECT POSTURE AND ALIGNMENT

Such sagging stretches the ligaments of your back and causes backache, etc. Ligaments that are unduly stretched are painful. Ligaments are meant to serve only as stops for the joints and they cannot be forcibly stretched without pain. When the ligaments in your back are made uncomfortable by stretching, it is only natural for your muscles to try to oppose the sagging of your back which results from the pull of gravity.

197

When your muscles are too weak to do their proper job, then they rapidly become exhausted and develop the terrible misery of fatigue, making your back even more uncomfortable. Check your symptoms! Do you notice a deep aching and soreness along the spine from stretched ligaments? Are your back and shoulder muscles achy and tired? Is your backache basically due to weak muscles? If it is, it's about time you did something sensible to relieve it, like strengthening those weak muscles by proper exercise.

Take the Mirror Posture Test

Look at yourself in the mirror. Do your shoulders slump? Is your upper back round? Do you have a potbelly? Are you a swayback? Can you now see the reasons why your back has the right to ache? The bending, slumping, ligament-stretching force of gravity has taken its toll. But even though you are presently a sufferer of backache due to weak muscles and bad posture, don't despair. You can restore back comfort with this posture exercise and The Bragg Healthy Lifestyle.

It has often been said that backache is the penalty man must pay for the privilege of standing and walking upright on two feet, often wearing uncomfortable shoes. Every infant struggles to stand instinctively on his own two feet and walk. He need not be taught. He will attempt this bipedal gait even if left alone most of the time and never instructed. It is natural for a human being to stand and walk in this manner. This is interesting, because there are no animals which spend all of their standing and walking hours on two feet, not even gorillas or chimpanzees. These apes use their hands and arms to help them move about. The world's strongest gorilla would be unable to follow a busy person, walking erectly, for more than a short time. This is because human beings are meant to walk erect and animals are not.

 198

Bragg Posture Exercise
Gives Instant Youthfulness

Before a mirror, stand up, feet 8" apart, stretch up spine. Tighten buttocks and suck in stomach muscles, lift up rib cage, put chest out, shoulders back, and chin up slightly. Line body up straight (nose plumbline straight to belly button), drop hands to sides and swing arms to normalize your posture. Do this posture exercise daily and miraculous changes will happen! You are retraining and strengthening your muscles to stand straight for health and youthfulness. Remember when you slump, you also cramp your precious machinery. This posture exercise will retrain your frame to sit, stand and walk tall for supreme health, fitness and longevity!

POSTURE CHART

	PERFECT	FAIR	POOR
HEAD			
SHOULDERS			
SPINE			
HIPS			
ANKLES			
NECK			
UPPER BACK			
TRUNK			
ABDOMEN			
LOWER BACK			

199

Your posture carries you through life from your head to your feet. This is your human vehicle and you are truly a miracle! Cherish, respect and protect you body by living The Bragg Healthy Lifestyle. – Patricia Bragg

Good Posture is Important For Health

The spines of human beings have natural curves which enable the muscles to oppose gravity and hold their backs erect. As long as the muscles are strong enough to maintain the balance of these curves and prevent back and shoulder sagging, the back is comfortable. When the muscles are too weak, the back sags, ligaments are stretched and backache results.

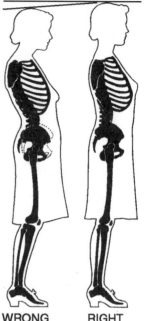

WRONG   RIGHT

To maintain oneself in a healthy state involves many factors: the right natural food, rest, exercise, sleep, fasting, control of emotions and mind and, last but not least, good posture. If a body is well-nourished and cared for, good posture is not a problem. When the body lacks the essentials, poor posture is often the result. Once poor habits have been established, one must faithfully each day practice corrective exercises and good posture habits.

How to Sit, Stand and Walk
For Strength, Youthfulness, Health

When walking, one should imagine that the legs are attached to the middle of the chest. That gives long, sweeping, graceful, springy steps because, when one walks correctly with this swing and spring, he automatically builds energy. Habit either makes or breaks us, and good posture habits make graceful, strong bodies. Just as the twig is bent, the tree is inclined.

When in a sitting position, see that the spine is stretched up and well back against the chair. Put shoulders back and lift chest up and off stomach, head high and never forward. Be sure to have both feet on the floor and never sit with your legs crossed. Under the knees run two of the largest arteries, carrying nourishing blood to the muscles below the knee and to the thousands of nerves that are found in the feet. When

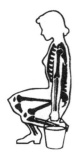
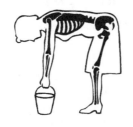
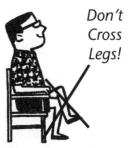

Don't Cross Legs!

Right way to lift   Wrong way to lift   Wrong way to sit!

you cross your legs you immediately cut down the blood to almost a trickle. When the muscles of the leg and knee are not nourished and do not have a good circulation, our blood goes stagnant in the extremities which can lead to varicose veins or broken capillaries. Look at the ankles of people over 40 who have made it a habit of crossing their legs and you'll see broken veins and capillaries. When the muscles and feet don't get their full supply of blood, the feet become weak and poor circulation sets in. Cold feet torment leg-crossers.

A well-known heart specialist was asked once, "When do most people have a heart attack?" The heart specialist answered, "At a time they are sitting quietly with one leg crossed over the other." So you can see that when you sit down, you should plant both of your feet squarely on the floor and never cross your legs. People who are habitual leg-crossers always have more acid crystals stored in the feet than those who never cross their legs while sitting. Crossing of the legs is one of the worst postural habits of man. It throws the hips, spine and the head off balance and can become one of the most insidious causes of a chronic backache. Poor posture of any kind can bring unbearable pain throughout the body, especially in the neck and lower back.

201

One very simple habit that is most beneficial to establish for your health is to stand, walk and sit tall and never sit with your legs crossed! Good posture does not require an exaggerated position. It's simply stretching up your spine and standing erect – which gives all your body's machinery room to operate and keep you healthier! When you maintain good posture, soon your body becomes more toned and healthier.

"The Illness That Cannot Be Cured By Fasting, Cannot Be Cured By Anything Else"

Dr. Nikolayev, director of a famous European fasting clinic, often quotes this old, wise German proverb above. Fasting permits the miracle cleansing and healing powers of the body, the mind and the soul to assert themselves.

Dr. Nikolayev – who fasts several times a year in 10 to 15 day stretches – stated, "I usually fast for health and spiritual reasons. I have also fasted several times for a scientific experiment. I always feel excellent when I fast. It is always a happy occasion and a good rest."

Dr. Nikolayev discovered his patients responded to fasting when all other forms of therapy had failed. The patients had been chronically ill and felt hopeless about their future! Most of them would never have functioned again. The famous doctor, Allan Cott, M.D. noted in his book *Fasting, The Ultimate Diet* (Bantam Books, NY) that 75% of those treated by fasting improved so remarkably that they were able to resume an active life!

Christian Century *magazine advised its readers to fast out of enlightened self-interest and with the objectives to improve health and make the body more vibrant and beautiful. "Fast because it is good for you," the magazine urged; it can be an "exercise to get the body in shape to be alive to itself. This process frees the self to be more sensitive to the Creation and to ourselves."*

Difficulties, like work are blessings in disguise. To the healthy man, difficulties should act as a tonic. They should open us to greater exertion. They should strengthen our willpower. – B.C. Forbes

Man is the sole and absolute master of his own fate forever. What he has sown in the times of his ignorance, he must inevitably reap; when he attains enlightenment, it is for him to sow what he chooses and reap accordingly. – Geraldine Coster

So we fasted and besought our God for this, and he listened to our entreaty. – Ezra 8:23

That fasting is a normal part of our walk with God is taken for granted by the Lord Jesus. Immediately following the Lord's Prayer, He said: "Moreover when ye fast . . . " – Matthew 6:16

Chapter 27

Doctor Human Mind

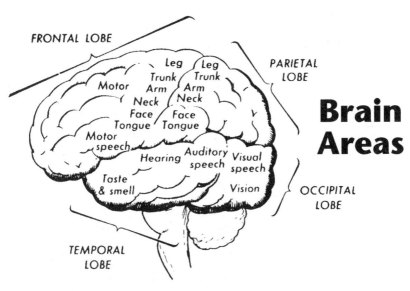

FRONTAL LOBE

PARIETAL LOBE

Leg Leg
Trunk Trunk
Motor Arm Arm
Neck Neck
Face Face
Tongue Tongue
Motor
speech
Hearing Auditory Visual
speech speech
Taste
& smell
Vision

Brain Areas

OCCIPITAL LOBE

TEMPORAL LOBE

203

There is an old German saying: "Alle gute Dinge sind Drei," or "All good things are three." We, as Christians worship a God represented by a trinity – the Father, Son and Holy Ghost. Man, too, is composed of a trinity. The **soul** is the first man, the ego, the individual, the personality, which makes each of us unique. The **mind** is the second man, through which the soul or the first man is expressed; the soul's only means of expression. The **body** is the third man, the physical, visible part; the means by which the mind expresses; also its only means, and its only mode of contact with environment. These three are one, just as the Godhead (Divine Force) is one, each making a part of this individual miracle called man.

Healthy Mind Habit:

Wake up and say - Today I am going to be happier, healthier and wiser in my daily living! I am the captain of my life and am going to steer it living a 100% healthy lifestyle! Fact – Happy people look younger and have fewer health problems! – Patricia Bragg

Your Body, Your Precious Home – Protect It

The body is composed of many members, yet is one body. If one of the members suffer, all others suffer with it. We recognize that the body is a whole, cannot be divided and is made up of a community of closely grouped and interrelated organs, tissues, and cells; each an individual unit, yet so closely related that not one of them can exist apart from the whole. For too long the public has viewed these various organs as unrelated, or loosely related, units. Most people are inclined to treat each more or less individually, not realizing that if one part of the indivisible whole suffers, all the rest suffer.

The body is the most wonderful miracle example ever created of widely diversified functions in one whole and it must be treated always as a unit. What is good for one part is good for all; what is bad is bad for all the parts.

If the toe is affected by gangrene, does not the whole body suffer with it? Not only is the pain inflicted on the whole man, but the absorption of decaying material has to be taken care of by the whole body – the loss of appetite, the headache, the nausea, the fever and the chills – yet the toe is the only affected member that can be seen. In the science of fasting, we are concerned with the whole person – including the soul, mind and body!

Correct Thinking is Important for Health

In the Book of Life, the Bible, Proverbs 23:7 tells us:
"For as he thinketh in his heart, so is he."
When a sick person constantly convinces himself that he will never get well, it becomes almost certain that his negativity and troubles will carry him to the grave.

Flesh is dumb! We never want you to forget that statement. That is the reason we use it over and over again. The mind, your computer, is really the controlling factor in your entire makeup. Flesh cannot think for itself because only the mind does all the thinking. That is why you must cultivate Positive Thinking.

Everything in excess is opposed by Nature.
– Hippocrates, the Father of Medicine

Your Mind Must Control Your Body!

The mind must have a will of iron and always be in command of the body. From this day forward learn how to substitute thoughts. When a negative thought – such as, "I am losing my energy because when you get older you start to lose energy" – enters your mind, replace it with positive thoughts that say, "Age cannot in any way affect my energy. Age is not toxic! I am ageless!"

Keep in mind always that whatever the mind tells the flesh, that is exactly what the flesh is going to believe and act upon. Your mind influences flesh. You must let your mind make decisions for your body, because if your body rules your mind, you face a life of misery and slavery!

Drugs Control Addict's Mind!

The "drug addict" is the extreme example of the body ruling the mind! This is why the world is over-populated with drug addicts. The body's craving for drugs is forcing the mind to command the body to commit crimes of violence so that it may satisfy the body with the drugs it craves. This is why the world is becoming crime riddled by drug addicts.

We maintain most of our bad habits simply because our minds are enslaved by our bodies. This applies also to alcohol, tea, coffee and other stimulants. The body rules by the false philosophy of "Eat, drink and be merry, for tomorrow we die." This is false. You don't die tomorrow, but if you continue to live by this wrong philosophy, 5, 10, 20 years later you will be burdened with a sick, prematurely aged body tormenting you daily!

Remember always that you are punished by your bad habits of living. Not *for* them, but *by* them! That is Mother Nature's Eternal Law. Sickness, aches, pains and physical suffering are ills that you are responsible for personally. You committed the crimes against your body because you did not use your God-given reason and intelligence to rule your body with your mind and live by natural laws.

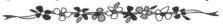

God gave His creatures light, air, & water open to the skies; man locks him in a stifling lair, then wonders why his brother dies. – Oliver Wendell Holmes

A Healthy Mind in a Healthy Body

What has your mind to do with health and long life? Far more than the majority of men and women realize! Think of your thoughts as powerful magnets, as entities which have the ability to attract or repel, according to the way they are used. A majority of people lean either to the positive or the negative side mentally. The positive phase is constructive and goes for success and positive achievements, while the negative side of life is destructive, leading to futility and failure. It's self-evident it's to our advantage to cultivate a positive healthy mental attitude. With patience, persistence and living The Bragg Healthy Lifestyle this can be accomplished.

There are many negative and destructive forms of thought which react in every cell in your body. The strongest is fear, and its child, worry – along with depression, anxiety, apprehension, jealousy, ill-will, envy, anger, resentment, vengefulness and self-pity. All of these negative thoughts bring tension to the body and mind leading to waste of energy, enervation and also slow or rapid poisoning of the body. Rage, intense fear and shock are very violent and quickly intoxicate the system. Worry and other destructive emotions act more slowly but, in the end, have the same destructive effect. Anger and intense fear stop digestive action, upset the kidneys and the colon causing total body upheaval (diarrhea or constipation, headaches, pains, fever, etc.).

Fear, worry and other destructive habits of thought muddle the mind! A crystal clear mind is needed to reason to your best advantage, enabling you to make sound, healthy decisions. An emotionally clouded mind often makes unwise and unhealthy decisions and might be unable to reach any positive conclusions at all!

What are the positive healthy mental forces or expressions? They are the ones that lead to peace of mind and inner relaxation, as opposed to the destructive habits which cause a tightening up of the entire system. This very second, let your mind take over your body.

Before you speak, always ask yourself – Is it good? Is it kind? Is it necessary?

Let Your Mind Guide You to Health!

In your mind, form an image of the person you want to be. Now, with Mother Nature's 9 Doctors as your helpers, you can make yourself exactly what you want to be! Believe in the power of positive thinking! Practice thought substitution. Never ever let a negative thought take over your mind. In this way, you set your own pattern of living and you make your mind a powerhouse of healthy, constructive thoughts. Strengthen your mind so thoroughly that if any weak, fearful relatives or friends tell you that fasting is starvation and that only harm can come from your health program . . . you can let their remarks slide out of your mind like water off a duck's back. You should feel sorry for these uninformed, fearful people because you will live to see many of them suffer and go to an early grave long before their time.

Miracle Rewards With Fasting:

- Each time you fast, your mind becomes stronger and more positive.
- Each time you fast, you will continue to eliminate fear, worry and other negative emotions.
- Fasting helps you spiritually. That is why Jesus, His followers and other spiritual leaders were fasters.
- Fasting elevates the soul, the mind and the body. What greater miracle rewards can you desire in life?

By fasting, you can create the person you have always desired to be. That is, you can if you demand and pursue only the best that life can offer!

Only when the body and mind are in harmony will there be opportunity for proper spiritual development; never forget that the spiritual man comes first, the mental is second and the physical is third. Only when the second and third aspects are in harmony can there be a proper balanced spiritual life!

Ten Little, Two-Letter Words Of Action To Say Daily:
If it is to be, it is up to me!

Inner Spiritual Harmony is Important

Spirituality depends far more on proper harmony of the rest of the man than is generally thought. We all have this power to create inner harmony through understanding the relationship of the body, mind and soul.

Use your mind to help you attain your desires by developing a constructive philosophy of life. Think constructively about health. Know the requirements of wholesome living and employ your determination, mind and willpower to live accordingly and to continue to do so. Health in soul, mind and body will be yours. Join hands with God and Mother Nature in making yourself a truly balanced, living trinity.

Fasting and The Bragg Healthy Lifestyle can take you to the heights of true living that few experience on this earth. Let your mind take control of your body this instant. New doors will open for you. You will be living in the light. Light is life, so let in the brightness of the light of a good and healthy life today!

208

Slow Me Down Lord

Slow me down Lord and fill me with your love.

Ease the pounding of my heart by the quieting of my mind.

Quiet my hurried pace with a vision of eternal time.

Give me, amid the confusion of the day,
    the calmness of the everlasting hills.

Break the tensions of my nerves and muscles with the soothing
    music of the singing streams that live in my memory.

Help me to know the magical, restoring power of sound sleep.

Teach me the art of taking minute vacations or slowing down
    to look at a flower, to chat with a friend, to pat a dog,
    to read a few lines from a good book.

Slow me down Lord and inspire me to send my roots deep
    into the soil of life's enduring values, so that I may
    grow toward the stars of my greater destiny.

Chapter 28

Spiritual Aspects of Fasting

As a crusader for the benefits of fasting for over 70 years, it is indeed gratifying to see the increased interest that has been developing in this subject during the past few decades. Not only has the medical profession rediscovered fasting as Mother Nature's primary method of healing and preventing sickness, but there is also a reawakening to the important role of fasting in attaining spiritual development.

My own regular program of fasting, as outlined in this book, is one of the main reasons that I am still alive! I'm blessed to see the fruition of our world health outreach to help make the world healthier. I am alert and ageless in body, mind and spirit as I approach the century mark.

During the first three quarters of the 20th century, I saw the world becoming more complex, chaotic and unhealthy. Most humans are feeling alienated, lost and confused. Most people are groping for stability in body, mind and soul in their hectic life.

In time of deep trouble, our natural instincts lead us back to the fundamentals of Mother Nature's Natural Laws. This return is usually made with knowledge gained from hard-learned lessons. Fasting as the means of purifying and healing body, mind and spirit is instinctive with animals, infants and among many cultures. Now we are beginning to learn the power of this simple, natural method. More books and articles are appearing that show the spiritual and physical benefits of fasting.

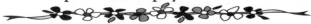

I humbled my soul with fasting. – Psalm 69:10

Your spiritual condition produces your physical condition. – Eph 4:1

*Is this not the fast I choose: to loose the bonds of wickedness,
to undo the thongs of the yoke, to let the oppressed go free
and to break every yoke? – Isaiah 58:6*

Fasting Gives Mental & Physical Awareness

As the body cleanses and heals itself through fasting, keener mental concentration and clearer spiritual perception develop. Remember, the brain is the physical instrument of the mind. As the mucus and toxic wastes are flushed from the brain cells, with it go the worries and frustrations from your mind. It becomes free and clear. You can then think intelligently and logically. Your memory becomes sharp and keen. Your creative powers are soon expanded. You are able to face reality and yourself . . . and begin to view your problems objectively to find definite answers – and solutions!

The elimination of toxic wastes releases the mind from physical bondage. The freedom from the bodily necessity of procuring, preparing, eating, digesting and assimilating food frees up and releases a tremendous amount of nervous energy which invigorates the mental and spiritual processes. You attain new levels of tranquillity, serenity and peace of mind. You become spiritually perceptive and receptive and at one with the Infinite. "Be still, and know that I am God."

"Fasting does not change God, but man. A cleansing process takes place. The awareness of the purification of the heart builds faith, and faith in God means authority with God." So stated Rev. Charles F. Stanley in an article on fasting in the *Moody Monthly*.

In *God's Chosen Fast* (Christian Literature Crusade, Ft. Washington, PA), author Arthur Wallis writes, "Without a doubt there is a very close connection between the practice of fasting and the receiving of spiritual revelation. Many non-Christian religions such as Buddhism, Hinduism, Confucianism and Islam also practice fasting because they know its power to detach one's mind from the world of sense, and to sharpen one's sensibility to the world of spirit."

If the stomach is full and busy, then the mind doesn't like to think.
– German Proverb

Every study in longevity shows that frugal eating promotes health and prolongs life. – Steve Meyerowitz, Juice Fasting and Detoxification

Great Spiritual Leaders Practiced Fasting

It was after fasting for 40 days and 40 nights that Moses received the Ten Commandments on Mount Sinai. Jesus spent 40 days and 40 nights fasting in the desert in preparation before starting His ministry.

The founders of the modern world's four major religions – Christianity, Judaism, Buddhism and Islam – taught fasting as a means of communication with the Divine through purification of body, mind and spirit. They instructed that fasting should be carried out with dedication and in private. Similar teachings are found in nearly all religions, ancient and tribal, as well as influential philosophies and moral codes. Zoroaster, the great Persian prophet, taught and practiced fasting. So did Plato, Socrates and Aristotle. Hippocrates, the Father of Medicine, considered fasting to be the great natural healer. The genius painter and sculptor Leonardo da Vinci also practiced and advocated fasting.

China's great philosopher and teacher, Confucius, included fasting in his precepts. The Yogis of India and Native Americans practice fasting as a means of spiritual enlightenment. The greatest modern example of the power of fasting is Mahatma Gandhi, who won India's freedom from the great British Empire in a complete and nonviolent victory of spiritual leadership.

211

My Unforgettable Experience with Gandhi

The date I met Gandhi was July 27, 1946 in New Delhi, which would become the capital of the new Republic of India a year and a month later. (India's independence became official on August 15, 1947.) At Gandhi's headquarters there, I received permission to accompany this amazing man on a 21 day fasting trip eastward through India's villages, where he would talk with the people and help them with their problems. At that time, the average Indian earned about 10 cents a day and starvation was a way of life. To show he shared their plight, this saintly and compassionate spiritual leader was planning to travel the dusty roads from village to village on foot, without food, only water; for 3 weeks.

Gandhi – A Spiritual Miracle

Gandhi was then 77 years of age and very frail in appearance. But his looks were indeed deceiving! This man was a tower of strength . . . physically, mentally and spiritually. His stamina, endurance, energy and mental abilities were astounding to everyone!

The trek began at sunup. The heat and humidity were the worst I have ever experienced. I have spent time in some of the hottest spots in the world, including Death Valley in California, the Sahara Desert and across North Africa on an 800 mile bicycle trip in intense summer heat. But never once did Gandhi seem to tire. Never once did he falter in his brisk pace of walking. The only time he sat down was during talks with the villagers. He would speak for 20 minutes, then answer questions for 20 minutes. Then we continued down the hot, dusty road to the next village. Gandhi ate nothing and drank only water flavored with lemon and honey.

Many who tried to travel with him fell by the wayside, suffering from heat and exhaustion. But Gandhi was inexhaustible. I have been an athlete and hiker all my life, but I have never seen anyone who had the physical stamina and energy as Gandhi. Each day he walked and talked until sundown before stopping for a rest. During the 21 day fasting walk, I had many talks with Gandhi on the power of fasting. Of all I learned from him, this statement seems to me the summation,

"All the vitality and energy I have comes to me because my body is purified by fasting." – Gandhi

Walking mile after mile from village to village, he gave the people courage and hope that a better life was coming to them. His internal strength and beautiful pure soul were so powerful that weak people felt strong after seeing him and hearing his wisdom. He gave his unlimited strength to the discouraged and the sick. He brought bright light and love where there was darkness.

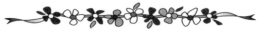

There is truth in the saying that man becomes what he eats. – Gandhi

Brisk walking is the king of exercise. With walking you discover the beauty of nature and it awakens and softens your soul and life! – Patricia Bragg

"Fasting Brings Spiritual Rebirth to All Who Cleanse and Purify Their Bodies."

Gandhi told the people to fast and purify their bodies and they would find peace and joy on earth. Gandhi said,

"The light of the world will illuminate within you when you fast and purify yourself."

This trip with the great Gandhi is an experience I will never forget! This physically small man was a spiritual giant. He led millions of people to independence from the mighty British Empire without striking a single physical blow. Yet, with all his power and influence, he was completely without arrogance. Characteristically, on the day of India's independence, Gandhi took no part in the celebrations that went on all over India; instead he spent the day in fasting and prayer in his garden.

The Grotto Where Jesus Fasted

On one of my trips to the Holy Land, I was in the area of Jericho. It was near the Mount of Temptation, where Jesus is said to have been tempted by the devil after his fast of 40 days and 40 nights. I decided to climb it. It was a long, easy ascent. From the top, which was still 200 feet below sea level, I looked down upon the hot, barren Jordan Valley.

On my descent, halfway down, I came upon a monastery built partly within the rock itself where 10 elderly Greek monks were living in poverty. Following the ancient custom of greeting any stranger as if he might be the wandering Christ, these monks welcomed me with beautiful courtesy. I was taken on a tour of the monastery. It was a fantastic place; parts of it jutted out over deep, brutal chasms while other rooms were carved out of the solid rock. One of these was a grotto which, my guide told me, was "the very spot where Jesus fasted 40 days and 40 nights, and was tempted by the devil."

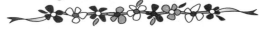

He fasted 40 days and 40 nights,
and afterward he was hungry. – Matthew 4:2

A soft answer turns away wrath, but harsh words cause quarrels.

The monks told me that they fasted 2 days every week, and once a year they fasted 40 days and nights in the grotto. They felt that this fasting had not only given them great spiritual enlightenment, but had also added many vigorous years to their lives.

Their appearance bore out their belief. Although far along in calendar years, these men had great flexibility in their bodies. It required a lot of physical stamina to keep the monastery in good condition in this rugged, barren wilderness and oven-like heat. All were lean and muscular, with the glow of health to their skin and bright, keen eyes – none of them wore glasses!

Their spiritual quality showed in the genuine brotherly love which they bestowed on me, a stranger. At the end of my visit, one of the monks escorted me to the gate, kissed me on both cheeks and gave me a blessing in Greek.

Looking back, as I descended the long, stony trail, I saw him watching solicitously. We waved to each other and I carried a warm glow of friendliness in my heart from that barren rocky land. Here again was proof of what I have learned from my own experience – that one of the spiritual benefits of fasting is a genuine sense of kinship and love for all humanity.

The Fast of 40 Days and 40 Nights

There is a significance to the "40 days and 40 nights" of fasting of the great spiritual leaders and of those who seek the highest spiritual enlightenment. This is the practical limit to which the disciplined body can exist without food before it begins to consume itself. The cleansing process has been completed, and all toxic wastes and excess fat have been "incinerated"– burned up into energy. When this limit is reached, starvation begins. The body will then have to feed on sound living tissue and this is harmful to body, mind and spirit. The fast should be terminated before this point is reached!

A long fast should not be attempted until the body has been trained to fast for short intervals, from 1 day up to 10 days, over a period of time.

The 40 days and 40 nights fast is not for the novice! It's only the experienced faster who learns to distinguish between the early cravings of habitual appetite and the warning pangs of genuine hunger.

At the beginning of a fast there is a craving for food which arises from the habit of eating at certain intervals. This may last for several days, but then the craving passes. There follows a short period of several days or more when the faster might feel some weakness and requires more rest. This is probably the most difficult part of the fasting experience.

Gradually this sense of weakness will disappear, signalling that the body has eliminated its worst wastes and poisons. Then comes a feeling of growing strength, with little or no concern about food, and an increasing mental alertness. There is a sense of release and freedom as one ascends to the higher levels of serenity and peace of mind. Spiritual awareness can reach a point of ecstasy!

How long this period lasts depends upon the individual. When the process of elimination of all wastes has been completed, the body signals a warning with pangs of genuine hunger. When this happens, whether in 2 to 4 weeks, the fast must end to preserve its benefits!

A Sound Mind in a Sound Body

Even the greatest spiritual leaders that the world has known trained themselves by habitual fasting, 1 or 2 days per week, before they undertook longer fasts. Herein lies the difference between genuine fasting and extreme asceticism, which has given fasting a bad name by prolonging it into starvation.

True fasting is psychosomatic (psycho – of the mind or spirit; and soma – of the body). It's truly a miracle natural means of achieving "a sound mind in a sound body," as the Greeks put it; or, according to the Bible,

"Your body is a temple of the Holy Spirit."

As I stride along on my daily two-mile brisk walk, I say to myself, often out loud, "Health, Strength, Youth, Vitality, Understanding, Joy, Peace and Salvation for Eternity!" It amazes me daily how our wonderful Lord fills my life with all His glorious blessings! – Patricia Bragg

Your Body is Your Temple
And Needs the Best Care

To quote again from Pastor Dr. Stanley, "According to medical experts, fasting is the most natural, original process of purifying the body. Since the Lord admonished man to work six days and rest one, would it not be equally wise to rest the digestive system for one day as well? I have found that fasting also sharpens the mind. The physical and spiritual benefits cannot be easily separated. A clear mind is essential to the desire for oneness and direction."

And from Arthur Wallis comes the observation that, "Our physical condition can often influence our spiritual lives more than we realize. Is God glorified when (our bodies) are weak or sickly through neglect of the divine laws that govern their well-being? Is God glorified when we become casualties from over-working, over-feeding or undernourishing our bodies, and failing to give them their 'Sabbath' of rest and relaxation? In an age of pressure, when the breakdown of mind or body is becoming all too familiar, the physical (as well as the spiritual) value of a fast of God's choosing becomes a matter of some importance. Here is a divine provision for health and healing, for renewal of mind and body, that we must further consider."

Courage, vitality, energy, endurance, zest and vigor are not mental states to be conjured up at will, but are the mental expression of a physical state. The Bible tells us that, "The kingdom of heaven is within." Fasting purifies all the trillions of cells of the body, including those of the brain. When the brain is free of toxic poisons the mind is liberated both psychologically and then spiritually. It's free from anxieties, boredom, loneliness, tension and fear. It can meet all of life's problems and make wise, better decisions. It can find more peace, joy and realize a fuller, more meaningful, healthier life.

Fasting is a natural tranquilizer with absolutely no negative side effects. A brain purified by fasting pays higher dividends than any other investment you can make. Begin today! Let this book be your guide and friend! Discover for yourself the Miracles of Fasting!

Take Time for 12 Things

1. Take time to **Work** –
   it is the price of success.
2. Take time to **Think** –
   it is the source of power.
3. Take time to **Play** –
   it is the secret of youth.
4. Take time to **Read** –
   it is the foundation of knowledge.
5. Take time to **Worship** –
   it is the highway of reverence and
   washes the dust of earth from our eyes.
6. Take time to **Help and Enjoy Friends** –
   it is the source of happiness.
7. Take time to **Love** –
   it is the one sacrament of life.
8. Take time to **Dream** –
   it hitches the soul to the stars.
9. Take time to **Laugh** –
   it is the singing that helps life's loads.
10. Take time for **Beauty** –
    it is everywhere in nature.
11. Take time for **Health** –
    it is the true wealth and treasure of life.
12. Take time to **Plan** –
    it is the secret of being able to have time
    for the first 11 things.

217

YOUR BIRTHRIGHT

HEALTH

CULTIVATE IT

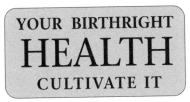

Have an
Apple
Healthy Day!

Teach me Thy way O Lord, and lead me in
a plain path. – Psalms 27:11

Exercise and Eat for Health

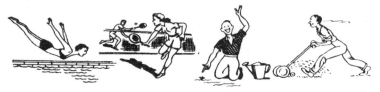

The Bragg Healthy Lifestyle
For a Lifetime of Super Health

In a broad sense, "The Bragg Healthy Lifestyle for the Total Person" is a combination of physical, mental, emotional, social and spiritual components. The ability of the individual to function effectively in his environment depends on how smoothly these components function as a whole. Of all the qualities that comprise an integrated personality, a totally healthy, fit body is one of the most desirable. Start today on your goals for more health, happiness and peace in your life.

A person is said to be totally physically fit if he functions as a total personality with efficiency and without pain or discomfort of any kind. This is to have a Painless, Tireless, and Ageless body. You possess sufficient muscular strength and endurance to maintain a healthy posture. You can successfully carry on the duties imposed by life and the environment, to meet any emergencies satisfactorily and have enough energy for recreation and social obligations after the "work day" has ended. You possess the body power (Vital Force) to recover rapidly from fatigue and stress of daily living without the aid of stimulants, drugs or alcohol. You can enjoy natural recharging sleep at night and awaken fit and alert in the morning for the challenges of the fresh new day ahead.

Keeping the body totally healthy and fit is not a job for the uninformed or the careless person. It requires an understanding of the body and of a healthy lifestyle and then following that lifestyle for a long, happy life. The purpose of "The Bragg Healthy Lifestyle" is to wake up the possibilities, a rebirth within you, of rejuvenation of your body, mind and soul for total, balanced body health. It's within your reach, so don't procrastinate, start today! Our hearts and prayers go out to touch your heart and soul with nourishing, caring love for your total health! With Love, Your Health Friends,

Patricia Bragg and Paul C. Bragg

Dear friend, I wish above all things that thou may prosper and be in health even as the soul prospers. – 3 John 2

Chapter 29

The Science of Eating For Super Health

It is the consensus of opinion among most people that we must eat, "To keep up our strength." This association of food and strength has been so driven into man's subconscious mind that he feels he must eat heavy, rich foods 3 times a day . . . "Something that sticks to the ribs." A person who has a big appetite they think of as a healthy person. If we know a person who has been sick, we are always encouraged when they're able to sit up and take nourishment.

During my long study and research into the value of food, I have come to regard nourishment as something more than habitual eating. The body can be fed with anything that is put into the stomach to subdue hunger. Food, however, plays an important role in our lives because the body is built from the food we eat. With food we either build strong, disease-free, youthful cells or we build sick cells . . . cells that do not support us as they should. So we must always eat food that builds sturdy, strong cells which are converted into healthy body tissue. We see a lot of people who are well-fed, but they are far from well-nourished! They have poor skin and muscle tone and lack energy, even though plenty of food is going into their bodies.

At one time in our early history, when our food came exclusively from Mother Nature, unprocessed and no toxic chemicals – we had a natural attraction to the kind of food our body needed. We had a superior sensitivity in our selection of food for life. In other words, there was an inner voice that told us what to eat. We can call it a God given instinct, that the animals in nature possess also. We were, in early times, naturally healthy, beautiful specimens as the Greeks and Romans used to be.

A Tropical Paradise For Health

I believe that man originated in the tropics, a natural paradise where his entire body was nourished by the gentle, healing rays of the sun. We know that the skin needs vitamin D, which is produced in response to sunshine. We also know that the skin needs vitamin A. But today man's body has become so degenerated, so filled with mucus, acid toxins, mineral and vitamin deficiencies that he can't spend a great amount of time in the sunshine. There are many people who develop all kinds of skin conditions from exposure to the sun and then falsely put the blame on sunshine. The sun pulls out the impurities below the skin – trying to purify you. Skin cancers spring from toxic cells. This is all the more reason to do your fasting/cleansing program!

Man has damaged his skin with the overuse of soap. I haven't used soap on my body for years, with the exception of washing my hands when water alone fails to remove the accumulated dirt.

I believe that in man's original home, the tropical paradise, his diet was made up of an abundance of raw fruits and vegetables, plus an abundance of all varieties of raw nuts and seeds. I believe that man was able to live for 900 years on this natural diet. His digestive system was perfectly attuned to his natural diet. Man, in his essential structure, has no weapons for killing. Therefore, I believe that the first people who inhabited the tropics of this earth were strictly vegetarians.

Today, humans live in air-conditioned, air-tight homes. We shut our bodies away from fresh air, breathing polluted air. We drink chemically treated water and do not get as much physical exercise as early humans enjoyed. The American man today has a life expectancy of 78 years, whereas men before the great flood may have lived for as long as 900 years. We have lost our tropical paradise. Man today lives in his poisoned cities, drinks his poisoned water, breathes polluted air and eats food that is grown in toxic soils, sprayed with poisons and picked half-ripe. Our living situations have changed dramatically, but we must do more than bemoan our lost Garden of Eden. We must face reality in all its ugliness.

Keep Healthy on the Alkaline Diet

Please understand that this program of eating is designed to give you the best nourishment that the food of civilization can offer you. At the same time, the suggested menus that follow are also for cleansing and purification. That is, you must look upon all organic fruits and vegetables not only as protective foods – not only as foods that are filled with minerals, vitamins, enzymes and valuable nutrients – but also as foods that are highly alkaline to help you keep your acidity down.

Many people studying nutrition become confused because there are so many opposing opinions. Some nutritionists advise a high-protein diet. Some nutritionists promote a low-carbohydrate diet. There are nutritionists who endorse a raw fruit, vegetarian or lacto-vegetarian diet. Each authority says that his is the best diet. I respect every scientist's views in the field of nutrition. He or she has come to these conclusions by study, research and observation. I believe that it is impossible to lay down absolute nutritional laws except when it comes to eliminating the dead, devitalized, demineralized, processed, sprayed and empty-calorie commercial foods of our present day civilization.

Today we have a selection of approximately 200 foods. You can build a healthy, delicious, adequate diet around these foods. As you fast and cleanse, you will purify your body. Also as you cleanse your body, your body itself will naturally make a selection of healthy foods.

The main thing is to eliminate the perverted foods of modern civilization. It is not so much a question of what you eat as what you shouldn't eat. On page 237 of this book I have given you the list of foods to avoid. There is an old cliche that says, "A man is either his own doctor at 40 or he is a fool." I must say here that I believe that any person 30 years of age who is not his own conscientious health captain is very soon going to run into some very serious physical problems!

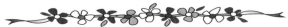

For the kingdom of God is not meat and drink; but righteousness, and peace and joy in the Creator. – Romans 14:17

Activity Draws on Your Vital Force's Energy

Our physical and mental activity draws heavily upon our Vital Force. Each of us has different demands. In my case, I push myself physically because I enjoy activity. I also enjoy mental activity. I like problems and enjoy the challenge of solving them. I don't live a soft life physically or mentally. As a man, I am a seeker for spiritual light, comfort, tranquillity and serenity. All of this takes my Vital Force's energy. Physical activity takes energy of one kind, mental tasks requires another and spiritual pursuits use another kind of energy.

One cannot give simple answers about nutrition. The nutritionist can give a lot of vital information, but she cannot eat for you or digest food for you or eliminate food for you. What I eat may not suit your needs, likes or dislikes. I don't eat as much food as the average person seems to crave and desire.

222

Every human is unique, as each snowflake is different. I am not trying to persuade you into fast changes. But if you want superior health you must eat a diet of simple, natural healthy foods. I am not going to tell you to be a raw food eater, a strict vegetarian, a lacto-vegetarian or a mixed eater. As you fast and as you purify your body, an inner voice, the natural instinct will gradually assert itself. I don't believe that you can quickly jump from a highly refined diet to a natural diet overnight of 60% raw fruits, veggies, whole grains, etc.

Mother Nature won't heal in sudden jolts. You ate in a certain pattern for many years, and your digestive and vital organs have adjusted themselves to this unhealthy diet. You have to move slowly. By body purification through fasting and adhering to the dictates of the 9 natural doctors, you will be enjoying the same super health as Patricia and I, plus millions of our followers. In time you will instinctively select natural, whole foods.

Every day the average heart, your best friend, beats 100,000 times and pumps 2,000 gallons of blood for nourishing your body. In 70 years that adds up to more than 360 million (faithful) heartbeats. Please be good to your heart and live The Bragg Healthy Lifestyle for a long, happy, healthy life!

Work Towards a Balanced, Natural Diet

You can't eat a nice, fresh combination health salad one day and the next day have a high fat, sugar, salt, refined, toxic food meal. Your nutrition has to be consistent. Let me illustrate what I mean. If you eat meat, I don't think you should eat it over 3 times a week. If you eat eggs, I don't think you should eat over 4 a week. If you drink milk, I think you should gradually eliminate it from your diet, along with all other dairy products. Man is the only creature that clings to milk after he has been weaned and the only creature that drinks the milk of another creature.

Building a good nutritional program is like climbing a ladder. There is the first rung – the elimination of all the devitalized, commercial, dead foods of civilization. That means the elimination of all unhealthy beverages – coffee, tea, alcohol and soft drinks. It means eliminating or reducing the amount of animal products, eggs and dairy products you eat daily. It means adding more raw organic fruits and vegetables to your diet until the total amount of raw foods is between 60% and 70% of your diet. As I stated earlier, when adding more fruits and vegetables to the diet, you have to slowly move with caution as you are deep house cleansing your body.

This period of discarding the devitalized foods of civilization and adding more raw fruits and vegetables to the diet is known as the cleansing "transition diet." Most people, from childhood until death, live on a diet that is predominantly on the acid side. This acid produces autointoxication and in turn, this toxic material causes aches, pains and degeneration of the body. So, if you have been living on a diet with mostly heavy cooked foods – such as meats, eggs, refined white breads, spaghetti, crackers and cookies, etc. – again let me warn you to slowly add more raw fruits and vegetables. After each weekly fast, you will be able to enjoy and want more raw fruits and raw vegetables in your diet, because fasting is purifying your body!

No milk available on the market today, in any part of the United States, is free of pesticide residues. – Info from a Congressional hearing

Eat Simple and Natural to Stay Healthy

After 3 months of faithfully fasting one day a week, you will be able to add at least 40% more raw fruits and vegetables to your diet. Remember these raw foods are the purifiers, cleansers and detoxifiers. These fruits and vegetables contain a lot of sunshine. They dig down into the old pockets of toxic poison and flush them out. This is how you can attain a superior state of Radiant Health! You are now going to keep internally clean and healthy.

People often ask at the Bragg Health Crusades, "Give me the perfect diet." This we cannot do because eating is such a personal nature . . . there are so many likes and dislikes that we can only counsel an individual through our books. We can only suggest that you reread and study the menus and food lists that we have included in this book so you can find foods that appeal to you and that will benefit your health.

Nutrition is like a chain in which all of the essential items are the separate links. If the chain is weak or is broken at any point the whole chain fails. If there are 40 items that are essential to the healthy diet, and one of these is missing, nutrition fails just as truly as it would if half the links were missing. The lack of any item (or several items) can result in ill health and even lead to death. An insufficient amount of any one item is enough to bring distress to the cells and tissues which are most vulnerable to this particular deficiency. It is not necessary that every item be furnished in required amounts at every meal, or every day, because our bodies always carry some reserves. As soon as the reserves are lost, be they large or small, they must be replenished.

Here are the healthy foods from which you can select when building your daily diet. You can divide your daily nutrition into one, two or three meals. As I have told you in this book, I do not eat breakfast, or if you call a bowl of fresh fruit a breakfast, then my breakfast is fresh fruit. I am not advising this practice for everyone; some people enjoy a large breakfast and a small lunch. Everyone's desires are different, but I feel that we don't need breakfast and I have explained my position fully.

Fruit – the Most Healthy Food for Man

I will start with the fresh fruit list since I regard fruit as the prize food of man. Fresh fruit or dried fruit can be used as a meal in itself, or it can be used as a dessert.

Organic Fruit – the Prize Food of Man

Apples	Kumquats
Apricots (fresh & dried)	Lemons & Limes
Avocados	Mangos
Bananas (fresh & dried)	Nectarines
Blueberries	Oranges
Cantaloupes	Papayas
Casaba Melon	Peaches
Cherries	Pears
Cranberries	Pineapples (fresh & dried)
Crenshaw Melon	Plums
Figs (fresh & dried)	Prunes (fresh & dried)
Grapefruits	Raspberries
Grapes (fresh & dried)	Strawberries
Honeydew Melon	Tomatoes
Kiwi	Watermelon

225

Note: Be sure dried fruits are unsulphured! Better yet, buy a dehydrator & make your own delicious dried fruit.

Raw, Unsalted Nut and Seed List

Nuts and seeds are rich in protein. You can select any 2 of the nuts and seeds when you are planning a meal. If you eat meat you still should not eat it over 3 times weekly, and on the other days you should eat the nuts or seeds for your protein. If you have tender gums or unreliable dentures, then you should purchase a coffee mill or small nut and seed grinding machine to make it easier to masticate, assimilate and digest nuts and seeds.

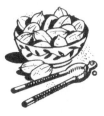

Almonds	Hazel Nuts
Brazil Nuts	Peanuts (Roasted)
Cashew Nuts	Pecans
Chestnuts	Pinones or Pine Nuts
Sesame Seeds	Sunflower Seeds
Filberts	Walnuts

Note: Most foods in this group are to be eaten raw and unsalted. It's best to buy nuts in their shells to maintain freshness.

Organic Vegetables – The Purifiers & Protectors

When planning your perfect health meals, you select the raw vegetables for your salad from this list. For the largest meal of the day, you should select 1 green and 1 yellow vegetable or you can select any other 2 vegetables from this list for your cooked vegetables:

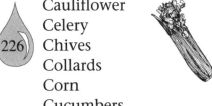

Alfalfa Sprouts
Artichokes
Jerusalem Artichokes
Asparagus
Beets
Bean Sprouts
Broccoli
Brussels Sprouts
Cabbages
Carrots
Cauliflower
Celery
Chives
Collards
Corn
Cucumbers
Dandelion Greens
Eggplant
Endive
Escarole
Garlic
Green Peas
Kale

Kohlrabi
Leeks
Lettuce
Mustard Greens
Okra
Onions
Oyster Plant
Parsnips
Peppers
Potatoes
Potatoes – sweet
Radishes
Shallots
Spinach
String Beans
Squash – many varieties
Swiss Chard
Tomatoes
Turnips
Turnip Greens
Wheat Grass
Watercress
Yams

Legumes

The legumes are one of man's oldest foods. They are healthy, hearty foods everyone can enjoy. They're rich in vegetable proteins, particularly soybeans. (See pg. 233)

Beans (all kinds)
Garbanzo Beans
Lentils

Lima Beans
Split Peas
Soybeans

If your enemy is hungry, give him food! If he is thirsty,
give him something to drink! – Proverbs 25:21

Natural Sweetening Agents

Although we have listed these natural sweetening agents, please remember that they still are highly concentrated foods and should be used sparingly.

Honey – raw, uncooked	Date Sugar – from dates
Pure Maple Syrup	Molasses – unsulphured
Evaporated Cane Juice	Blackstrap Molasses
Barley Malt, Rice Syrup	Concentrated Fruit Juices

Natural Oils

These oils are unsaturated and allowable, but use sparingly. Read labels: refuse oils that contain harsh chemicals to prevent rancidity. Cold-pressed or expeller-pressed oils from health stores are the best.

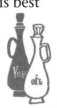

Olive Oil – virgin is best	Corn Oil
Hempseed Oil	Sesame Seed Oil
Safflower Oil	Walnut Oil
Soy Oil	Flaxseed Oil
Sunflower Oil	Peanut Oil
Avocado Oil	Almond Oil

227

Natural Whole Grains, Flours & Cereals

These 100% whole grains are best for your health. Use for cooking, bread and pastry baking and with cereals. Cereals should not be eaten more than 3 times a week unless you do heavy physical labor or heavy sports training. On your cereal you can use any of the natural sweetening agents and Rice Dream, almond or soy milks.

Whole Wheat, unbleached	Rye
Whole Barley	Flax
Millet	Quinoa
Corn Meal -Yellow, White & Blue	Amaranth
Oats - steel cut oats (a Bragg favorite)	Buckwheat
Brown Rice - all natural & unrefined	Bulgur

rices are good – long & short grain, Basmati & wild rice.

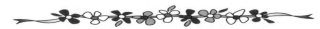

The body is the soul's house. Shouldn't we take care of our house so that it doesn't fall into ruin? – Philo, Alexandrian philosopher

For those used to 3 meals daily – here's some suggestions:

Suggestion # 1:   Breakfast

After exercise, stretching, etc. have the Bragg Pep Drink or a dish of fresh fruit. Optional, hot or cold whole grain bran cereal with a sliced banana as topping, sweetened with honey or maple syrup and add Rice Dream or soy milk if desired. Herbal tea sweetened with honey (optional).

Lunch

A raw veggie salad. Bowl of veggie soup. Fresh fruit for dessert.

Dinner

Raw vegetable salad. Choice of vegetable protein, beans, tempeh, soy, tofu. Two cooked vegetables. Fresh fruit for dessert and a whole grain cookie or health pastry.

Suggestion # 2:   Breakfast

Bragg Pep Drink. Fresh or unsulphured stewed fruit. One fresh, fertile egg, two slices of whole grain toast (you may enjoy whole grain or blue corn pancakes or waffles occasionally).

Lunch

Variety raw vegetable salad, soup or vegetarian casserole, steamed zucchini or yellow squash. Fresh fruit for dessert.

Dinner

Raw vegetable salad. Salad and dressing recipe on page 231. Use salad dressing sparingly and keep in refrigerator. Green peppers stuffed with brown rice and tofu. Choice of cooked fresh vegetable. Fresh fruit and 2 dates for dessert.

Suggestion # 3:   Breakfast

Bragg Pep Drink. Optional with whole grain bran muffin. We prefer our Pep Drink for breakfast – it's super for energy and nutrition and doesn't overload your digestive system!

Lunch

Raw variety vegetable salad, corn on the cob or brown rice and lentil casserole. Fresh fruit for dessert.

Dinner

Raw vegetable or fresh fruit salad. A vegetable protein dish. Baked eggplant, bowl of mustard greens and stewed tomatoes. Fresh fruit for dessert or whole grain crust apple pie.

Enjoy a Large Variety of Wholesome, Natural, Delicious and Nutritious Foods

Here are 200 foods that we have listed as good natural foods to eat and create your menus from. It is our recommendation you go over this list of foods, see what you like and build your menus to suit yourself and your family. Also, be brave and try new healthy foods.

People have built up such strong desires for certain foods that they think it's impossible for them to give up those foods. We are talking about healthy foods that appear on these lists, not the devitalized foods. The Bible tells us that God provided an ideal diet in the Garden of Eden. It plainly states, "And God said . . .

" I give you every seed-bearing plant on the face of the whole earth, and every tree that has fruit with seed in it. They will be yours for food."

– Genesis 1:29, *Holy Bible, NIV*

In other words, God gave man fruits, vegetables, nuts, seeds and grains for a diet that would give health and long life. We read in the Bible that people who ate this diet lived as many as 900 years. If man lived on the simple foods of Mother Nature, he experienced superior health and freedom from all ailments and a long life.

Over the years man started changing, processing and refining his natural food. Many foods which he now eats are dead, foodless foods. The further man strayed away from his natural foods, the more trouble he got into. As long as he lived on an abundance of raw fruits and vegetables, properly cooked vegetables and the raw unsalted nuts and seeds, he enjoyed a longer life and vitality supreme. Natural foods are the only foods that promote higher health. These are the foods that our digestive system was made to handle and process for keeping us healthy.

The more natural you make your diet, the better health you are going to have! You have 200 foods here to select from. With these foods and your program of fasting, there is no reason why you shouldn't keep in prime physical condition at all times!

These freshly squeezed organic vegetable and fruit juices are important to The Bragg Healthy Lifestyle. It's not wise to drink beverages with your main meals, as it dilutes the digestive juices. But it's great during the day to have a glass of freshly squeezed orange, grapefruit, vegetable juice, Bragg Vinegar Drink, herb tea or try a hot cup of Bragg Liquid Aminos Broth (½ to 1 tsp Bragg Liquid Aminos in cup of hot distilled water) – these are all ideal pick-me-up beverages.

Bragg Apple Cider Vinegar Drink– Mix 1-2 tsp. equally of Bragg Organic ACV and (optional) raw honey or pure maple syrup in distilled water. Take 1 glass upon arising, an hour before lunch and dinner.

Delicious Hot Cider Drink – Add a few cinnamon sticks and cloves to hot distilled water and let steep for 20 mins. Before drinking add 2 tsps Bragg Raw Organic Apple Cider Vinegar and raw honey equally.

Bragg Favorite Juice Cocktail – This drink consists of all raw vegetables (please remember organic is best) which we prepare in our vegetable juicer: carrots, celery, beets, cabbage, watercress and parsley. The great purifier, garlic we enjoy, but it's optional.

Bragg Favorite Healthy "Pep" Drink – After our morning stretch and exercises we enjoy this instead of fruit. It's also delicious and powerfully nutritious as a meal anytime: lunch, dinner or take along in a thermos to work, picnics, school, the gym, or on your nature walks, etc.

230

Bragg Healthy Pep Drink

Prepare the following in blender, add 1 ice cube if desired colder:
Choice of: freshly squeezed orange juice, grapefruit or tangelo; carrot and greens juice; unsweetened pineapple juice; or 1 ½ cups distilled water with:

½ tsp raw wheat germ	*¼ tsp vitamin C powder*
⅓ tsp flaxseed oil, optional	*¼ tsp nutritional yeast flakes*
¼ tsp green powder (barley, etc.)	*1 to 2 bananas, ripe*
½ tsp raw oat bran	*1 tsp raw honey, optional*
½ tsp psyllium husk powder	*1 tsp soy protein powder*
½ tsp lecithin granules	*1 tsp raw sunflower seeds*

Optional: 4 apricots (sun dried, unsulphured). Soak in jar overnight in distilled water or unsweetened pineapple juice. We soak enough to last for several days. Keep refrigerated. In summer, you can add fresh fruit in season: peaches, strawberries, berries, apricots, etc. instead of the banana. In winter, add apples, kiwi, oranges, pears or persimmons or try sugar-free, frozen organic fruits. Serves 1 to 2.

Patricia's Delicious Health Popcorn

Use freshly popped popcorn (I prefer air popped). If desired, use olive, soy, or safflower oil or melted salt-free butter. Sparingly pour oil over popcorn and add several sprays of Bragg Liquid Aminos and Apple Cider Vinegar. Sprinkle with nutritional yeast large flakes. For variety, try: pinch of Italian or French herbs, cayenne pepper, mustard powder or fresh crushed garlic to the oil mixture. Delicious served instead of breads!

Bragg's Lentil & Brown Rice Casserole

14 oz pkg lentils, uncooked
4 carrots, chopped
3 celery stalks, chopped
2 onions, chopped
3 quarts distilled water

4 garlic cloves, chopped
1 cup brown rice, uncooked
1 tsp Bragg Liquid Aminos
¼ tsp Italian herbs (oregano, basil, etc.)
2 tsp olive oil (virgin - cold-pressed is best)

Wash & drain lentils and rice. Place grains in large stainless steel pot. Add water. Bring to boil, reduce heat, simmer for 30 minutes. Then add vegetables & seasonings to rice & cook on low heat until done. Just before serving, add fresh or canned tomatoes. For a delicious garnish add parsley & nutritional yeast large flakes. Add more water in cooking the grains to make a delicious soup or stew. Serves 4 to 6.

Bragg Raw Vegetable Health Salad

2 stalks celery, chopped
1 bell pepper & seeds, diced
½ cucumber, chopped
1 carrot, grated
1 raw beet, grated
1 cup green cabbage, sliced

½ cup red cabbage, chopped
½ cup alfalfa or sunflower sprouts
2 spring onions & tops, chopped
1 turnip, grated
1 avocado (ripe)
3 tomatoes, medium size

For variety add raw zucchini, sugar peas, mushrooms, broccoli, cauliflower. Dice avocado & tomato and serve on side as a dressing. Chop, slice or grate vegetables fine to medium for variety in size. Mix vegetables thoroughly & serve on a bed of lettuce, spinach, watercress or chopped cabbage. Serve choice of fresh squeezed lemon, orange or dressing separately. Chill salad plates before serving. Always eat salad first before serving hot dishes. Serves 3 to 5.

231

Bragg Vinaigrette Health Dressing

½ cup Bragg Apple Cider Vinegar
2 tsps raw honey
⅓ cup virgin olive oil, or blend with safflower, soy, sesame or flax.
1 Tbsp fresh herbs, minced or pinch of Italian or French dry herbs

⅓ tsp Bragg Liquid Aminos
1 to 2 cloves garlic, minced

Blend ingredients in blender or jar. Refrigerate in covered jar.

For delicious herbal vinegar: in quart jar add ⅓ cup tightly packed, crushed fresh sweet basil, tarragon, dill, oregano, or any fresh herbs desired, combined or singly. (If *dried* herbs, use 1 to 2 tsp. herbs.) Now cover to top with Bragg Organic Raw Apple Cider Vinegar and store 2 weeks in warm place, strain and refrigerate.

Honey-Celery Seed Vinaigrette

¼ tsp dry mustard
¼ tsp Bragg Liquid Aminos
¼ tsp paprika
3 Tbsp raw honey

1 cup Bragg Apple Cider Vinegar
½ cup virgin olive oil
1 medium onion, minced
⅓ tsp celery seed

Blend ingredients in blender or jar. Refrigerate in covered jar.

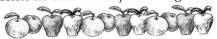

Food and Product Summary

Today, many foods are highly processed or refined, which robs them of essential nutrients, vitamins, minerals and enzymes. Many contain harmful chemicals. The research findings of top nutritionists, physicians and dentists have led to the discovery that devitalized foods are the major cause of poor health, illness, dental problems, cancer and premature death. The huge increase in the last 70 years of degenerative diseases such as heart disease and arthritis substantiate this. Scientific research has shown that most of these afflictions can be prevented and that others, once established, may be arrested or even reversed through nutritional methods.

Enjoy Super Health with Natural Foods

1. **RAW FOODS:** Use fresh fruits and raw vegetables, the organically grown are always best. Enjoy nutritious variety garden salads with sprouts and raw nuts and seeds.

2. **VEGETABLE and ANIMAL PROTEINS:**
   a. Legumes, lentils, brown rice, soy beans, beans.
   b. Nuts and seeds, raw and unsalted.
   c. Animal protein (if you must) – hormone free meats, liver, kidney, brain, heart, poultry, seafood. Please eat these proteins sparingly or it's best to enjoy the healthier vegetarian diet. You can bake, roast, wok or broil these proteins. Eat meat no more than 3 times a week.
   d. Dairy products – eggs (fertile, fresh), unprocessed hard cheese, goat's cheese and certified raw milk. We choose not to use dairy products. Try the healthier soy, nut (almond, etc.) and Rice Dream – the non-dairy milks.

3. **FRUITS and VEGETABLES:** Organically grown is always best – grown without the use of poisonous sprays and toxic chemical fertilizers whenever possible; ask your market to stock organic produce. Steam, bake, saute or wok veggies for as short a time as possible to retain the best nutritional content and flavor. Also enjoy fresh juices.

4. **100% WHOLE GRAIN CEREALS, BREADS and FLOURS:** They contain important B-complex vitamins, vitamin E, minerals and the important unsaturated fatty acids.

5. **COLD or EXPELLER-PRESSED VEGETABLE OILS:** Virgin olive oil, soy, sunflower, flax and sesame oils are excellent sources of healthy, essential, unsaturated fatty acids; but it's still wise to use all oils sparingly.

232

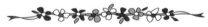

Healthy, organic foods have a wonderful abundance of potential life energy.

Vegetable Protein Percentage Chart

LEGUMES %

	%
Soybean sprouts	54
Mungbean sprouts	43
Soybean curd (tofu)	43
Soy flour	35
Soybeans	35
Soy sauce	33
Broad beans	32
Lentils	29
Split peas	28
Kidney beans	26
Navy beans	26
Lima beans	26
Garbanzo beans	23

VEGETABLES %

	%
Spinach	49
New Zealand Spinach	47
Watercress	46
Kale	45
Broccoli	45
Brussels Sprouts	44
Turnip Greens	43
Collards	43
Cauliflower	40
Mustard Greens	39
Mushrooms	38
Chinese Cabbage	34
Parsley	34
Lettuce	34
Green Peas	30
Zucchini	28
Green beans	26
Cucumbers	24
Dandelion Greens	24
Green Pepper	22
Artichokes	22
Cabbage	22
Celery	21
Eggplant	21
Tomatoes	18
Onions	16
Beets	15
Pumpkin	12
Potatoes	11
Yams	8
Sweet Potatoes	6

GRAINS %

	%
Wheat germ	31
Rye	20
Wheat, hard red	17
Wild rice	16
Buckwheat	15
Oatmeal	15
Millet	12
Barley	11
Brown rice:	8

FRUITS %

	%
Lemons	16
Honeydew melon	10
Cantaloupe	9
Strawberry	8
Orange	8
Blackberry	8
Cherry	8
Apricot	8
Grape	8
Watermelon	8
Tangerine	7
Papaya	6
Peach	6
Pear	5
Banana	5
Grapefruit	5
Pineapple	3
Apple	1

NUTS AND SEEDS %

	%
Pumpkin seeds	21
Sunflower seeds	17
Walnuts, black	13
Sesame seeds	13
Almonds	12
Cashews	12
Filberts	8

233

Data obtained from *Nutritive Value of American Foods in Common Units,* USDA Agriculture Handbook No. 456. Reprinted with author's permission, from *Diet for a New America* by John Robbins (Walpole, NH: Stillpoint Publishing).

Healthy Foods Naturally Vitamin E Rich Are Important for Your Health

This is a list of foods that contain the following notable amounts of precious, healthy Vitamin E. This list was compiled from *Bridges Food and Beverage Analyses*.

Food	Quantity	Vitamin E IU's
Apples	1 medium	0.74
Bananas	1 medium	0.40
Barley	½ cup	4.20
Beans, Navy	½ cup	3.60
Butter (salt-free)	6 tablespoons	2.40
Carrots	1 cup	0.45
Celery, Green	½ cup	2.60
Corn, Dried for Popcorn	1 cup	20.00
Cornmeal, Yellow	½ cup	1.70
Corn Oil	6 tablespoons	87.00
Eggs, Fertile	2	2.00
Endive, Escarole	½ cup	2.00
Flour, Whole grain	1 cup	54.00
Grapefruit	½	0.52
Kale	½ cup	8.00
Lettuce	6 leaves	0.50
Oatmeal	½ cup	2.00
Olive Oil (virgin)	½ cup	5.00
Onions, Raw	2 medium	0.26
Oranges	1 small	0.24
Parsley	½ cup	5.50
Peas, Green	1 cup	4.00
Potatoes, White	1 medium	0.06
Potatoes, Sweet	1 small	4.00
Rice, Brown	1 cup cooked	2.40
Rye	½ cup	3.00
Soybean Oil	6 tablespoons	140.00
Sunflower Seeds, Raw	½ cup	31.00
Wheatgerm Oil	6 tablespoons	50 – 420.00

The Bragg Gourmet Health Recipe Book (448 pages) – there's 54 Healthy Salad Recipes & 23 Dressing Recipes. *See back pages for booklist.*

A recent revealing study of nurses whose daily Vitamin E intake was 100 mgs and more had a 36% lower risk of heart attack and 23% lower risk of stroke.

Phytochemicals - Nature's Miracles Help Prevent Cancer

Make sure to get your daily dose of these naturally occurring, cancer-fighting biological substances that are abundant in onions, garlic, beans, legumes, soybeans, cabbage, cauliflower, broccoli, citrus fruits, etc. The champion is the tomato, which contains about 10,000 different phytochemicals!

Class	Food Sources	Action
PHYTOESTROGENS	Soy products, alfalfa sprouts, red clover sprouts, licorice root (not candy)	May block some cancers, & aids in menopausal symptoms
PHYTOSTEROLS	Plant oils, corn, soy, sesame, safflower, wheat, pumpkin	Blocks hormonal role in cancers, inhibits uptake of cholesterol from diet
SAPONINS	Yams, beets, beans, nuts, soybeans	May prevent cancer cells from multiplying
TERPENES	Carrots, yams, winter squash, sweet potatoes, apricots, cantaloupes	Antioxidants – protects DNA from free radical-induced damage
	Tomatoes and tomato-based products	Helps block UVA & UVB & may help protect against prostate cancers, etc.
	Citrus fruits (flavonoids)	Promotes protective enzymes; antiseptic
	Spinach, kale, beet & turnip greens	Protects eyes from macular degeneration
	Red chile peppers	Keeps carcinogens from binding to DNA
PHENOLS	Fennel, parsley, carrots, alfalfa	Prevents blood clotting & may have anticancer properties
	Citrus fruits, broccoli, cabbage, cucumbers, green peppers, tomatoes	Antioxidants – flavonoids block membrane receptor sites for certain hormones
	Grape seeds	Strong antioxidants; fights germs & bacteria, strengthens immune system, veins & capillaries
	Grapes, especially skins	Antioxidant, antimutagen; promotes detoxification. Acts as carcinogen inhibitors
	Yellow & green squash	Antihepatoxic, antitumor
SULFUR COMPOUNDS	Onions & garlic (fresh is best)	Promotes liver enzymes, inhibits cholesterol synthesis, reduces triglycerides, lowers blood pressure, improves immune response, fights infections, germs & parasites

Body Signs of Potassium Deficiency

🍎 Bone and muscle aches and pains, especially lower back.

🍎 Shooting pains when straightening up after leaning over.

🍎 Dizziness upon straightening up after leaning over.

🍎 Morning dull headaches upon arising and when stressed.

🍎 The body feels heavy, tired and it's an effort to move.

🍎 Dull, faded-looking hair that lacks sheen and luster.

🍎 The scalp is itchy. Dandruff, premature hair thinning or balding may occur.

🍎 The hair is unmanageable, mats, often looks straw-like, is sometimes extremely dry and other times oily.

🍎 The eyes itch, feel sore and uncomfortable, and appear bloodshot and watery. Also, eyelids may be granulated with white matter collecting in the corners.

236

🍎 The eyes tire easily and will not focus as they should.

🍎 Loss of mental alertness and onset of confusion, making decisions difficult. The memory fails, making you forget names and places you should remember.

🍎 You tire physically and mentally with the slightest effort.

🍎 You become easily irritable and impatient with your family, friends and loved ones, and even with your business and social acquaintances.

🍎 You feel nervous, depressed and in a mental fog. You have difficulty getting things done, due to mental and muscle fatigue. The slightest effort can leave you upset and trembling.

🍎 At times, your hands and feet get chilled, even in warm weather, which is a sign of potassium deficiency.

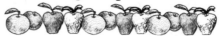

Potassium is the key mineral in the constellation of minerals; it's so important to every living thing that without it there would be no life. Raw apple cider vinegar is a rich source of potassium.

Avoid These Processed, Refined, Harmful Foods

Once you realize the harm caused to your body by refined, chemicalized, deficient foods, you'll want to eliminate these "killer" foods. Follow The Bragg Healthy Lifestyle for it provides the basic, essential nourishment your body needs to maintain long-lasting health.

- Refined sugar or refined sugar products such as jams, jellies, preserves, marmalades, yogurts, ice cream, sherbets, Jello, cake, candy, cookies, chewing gum, soft drinks, pies, pastries, tapioca puddings and all sugared fruit juices and fruits canned in sugar syrup. (Health stores have healthy, delicious replacements, so seek, buy and enjoy!)

- White flour products such as white bread, wheat-white bread, enriched flours, rye bread that has white flour in it, dumplings, biscuits, buns, gravy, pasta, pancakes, waffles, soda crackers, pizza, ravioli, pies, pastries, cakes, cookies, prepared and commercial puddings and ready-mix bakery products. (Health Stores have a huge variety of 100% whole grain products – delicious breads, crackers, pastas, pizzas, pastries, etc.)

- Salted foods, such as corn chips and potato chips, crackers and nuts.

- White rice and pearled barley.   • Fried and greasy foods.

- Commercial, hi-processed dry cereals made from corn, oats, etc.

- Food that contains palm and cottonseed oil. Products labeled vegetable oil . . . find out what kind before you use them.

- Peanuts and peanut butter that contains hydrogenated, hardened oils and any mold that can cause allergies.

- Margarine – full of dangerous, unnatural, trans-fatty acids.

- Saturated fats and hydrogenated oils – enemies that clog the arteries.

- Coffee, decaffeinated coffee, China black tea and all alcoholic beverages. Also all caffeinated and sugared cola and soft drinks.

- Fresh pork and pork products.   • Fried, fatty and greasy meats.

- Smoked meats, such as ham, bacon, sausage and smoked fish.

- Luncheon meats, hot dogs, salami, bologna, corned beef, pastrami and packaged meats containing dangerous sodium nitrate or nitrite.

- Dried fruits containing sulphur dioxide – a toxic preservative.

- Don't eat chickens or turkeys that have been injected with stilbestrol or fed with commercial poultry feed containing any drugs or toxins.

- Canned soups - read labels for sugar, starch, flour and preservatives.

- Food that contains benzoate of soda, salt, sugar, cream of tartar . . . and any other additives, drugs or preservatives.

- Day-old cooked vegetables, potatoes and pre-mixed, wilted salads.

- Pasteurized, filtered vinegars, distilled white, malt and synthetic vinegars – these are the dead vinegars! (We use only organic, raw, unfiltered apple cider vinegar with the "mother" as used in olden times.)

237

THE MIRACLES OF APPLE CIDER VINEGAR FOR A STRONGER, LONGER, HEALTHIER LIFE

The old adage is true:
"An apple a day helps keep the doctor away."

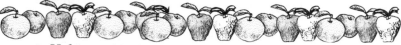

- Helps maintain a youthful, vibrant body
- Helps fight germs and bacteria naturally
- Helps retard the onset of old age in humans, pets and farm animals
- Helps regulate calcium metabolism
- Helps keep blood the right consistency
- Helps regulate women's menstruation
- Helps normalize the urine, thus relieving the frequent urge to urinate
- Helps digestion and assimilation
- Helps relieve sore throats, laryngitis and throat tickles and cleans out toxins
- Helps sinus, asthma and flu sufferers to breathe easier and more normally
- Helps maintain healthy skin, soothes sunburn
- Helps prevent itching scalp, dry hair and baldness, and banishes dandruff
- Helps fight arthritis and removes crystals and toxins from joints, tissues and organs
- Helps control and normalize weight

– Paul C. Bragg, Health Crusader,
Originator of Health Stores

Our sincere blessings to you, dear friends, who make our lives so worthwhile and fulfilled by reading our teachings on natural living as our Creator laid down for us to follow. He wants us to follow the simple path of natural living. This is what we teach in our books and health crusades worldwide. Our prayers reach out to you and your loved ones for the best in health and happiness. We must follow the laws He has laid down for us, so we can reap this precious health physically, mentally, emotionally and spiritually!

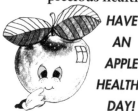

**HAVE
AN
APPLE
HEALTHY
DAY!**

With Love,

Patricia Bragg

Organic Raw Apple Cider Vinegar with the "Mother" is the #1 food I recommend to maintain the body's vital acid-alkaline balance.
– Gabriel Cousens, M.D., Author, *Conscious Eating*

238

Chapter 30

Mother Nature Knows No Mercy

There is no thought or discrimination in the working of the Eternal Laws that govern all things. Evenly, ruthlessly, eternally, Mother Nature works according to fixed laws for good or for ill . . . thinking as little of us creatures that build and die on this earth as the boy at play thinks of the ant hill beneath his foot.

It is for the ant to select a safe, secluded place for her nest, or suffer the consequences. It is for us to study Mother Nature's Eternal Laws, and adjust ourselves to them, or suffer. Mother Nature has no time or thought for individual cases! Fire will burn the innocent child and spare the hardened criminal who knows the ways of fire. It is well for us that it is so, for our real education is acquired by the study of the Natural Laws that will not coddle or spare us.

239

Mother Nature is unsentimental and powerful in her work on this earth – disregarding man's sense of justice or injustice! She may crush the just man and his family who disobey her Eternal Laws with disease and premature ageing, yet spares the criminal who follows the natural plan of physical health.

The purpose of this book is to help you save yourself by following the Natural Laws of Living. Follow The Bragg Healthy Lifestyle which are the laws of natural living and you will save yourself from needless suffering. You can achieve supreme health to live a long, vital life.

E. M. Forster, one of Britain's literary immortals, observed that food is one of the five main facts of life, "a link between the known and the forgotten." It was a marvel to him that we continually – "day after day put an assortment of objects into a hole in our faces without becoming surprised or bored."

In the course of a year, the average adult eats 133 pounds of sugar, 53 pounds of fats, 100 pounds of white flour, 14 pounds of white rice, 25 pounds of potatoes, and often quarts of ice cream. There can be no arguing that many mouths function as litter baskets and garbage dumps.

Mother Nature Wants Us Clean & Healthy

Mother Nature tells us we must keep clean inside and not allow toxic poisons, obstructions, water and morbid poisons to accumulate within our bodies. A regular fasting program as given in this book teaches you the great Law of Internal Purity.

Self-preservation is the first Law of Life. If we are to live a long, healthy, active, happy life, we must work with Mother Nature and not against her! If you attempt to break her laws she will break you! Natural laws are God's Good Laws. If we follow them, we will be rewarded with Super Health! Mother Nature's strict laws demand you keep your body clean inside and there's no better way to keep yourself clean internally than by fasting!

Make Mother Nature your personal friend. Here is a friend that will never fail you, if you will work with her and not against her. If, after reading this book, it sounds reasonable and intelligent – follow it. Live by it and let no man keep you away from living by the Natural Laws.

240

Which Kind of Person are You?

There are only 2 kinds of people in the world. Which kind are you? The real person thinks for himself. The imitation person lets others think for him!

It takes courage to live your own life. Fasting and living the Healthy Life takes courage in this sick, poisoned world. Set a high standard of living for yourself. Demand the best health! Let no weakling drag you down to his level. It is the survival of the fittest. Be fit! Be strong! Live long, happy and with vigor!

Let this book be your guide and mentor to a healthy life. May the knowledge and wisdom in this book bring you a new healthy life filled with fresh youthful energy, peace of mind and the joy of living.

Everyone should be his own physician. We ought to assist and not force nature. – Voltaire

Pure water is the cheapest form of medicine to a dehydrated body.
– F. Batmanghelidj, M.D.,
Your Body's Many Cries for Water; You Are Not Sick, You Are Thirsty.

Alternative Health Therapies And Massage Techniques

Explore these wonderful natural methods of healing your body. Then choose the technique best for you:

Acupuncture/Acupressure – Acupuncture directs and rechannels body energy by inserting hair-thin needles (use only disposable needles) at specific points on the body. It's used for pain, backaches, migraines and general body disfunction. Used in Asia for centuries, acupuncture is safe, virtually painless and has no side effects. Acupressure is based on the same principles and uses finger pressure and massage rather than needles.

Chiropractic – Daniel David Palmer founded chiropractic in 1885 in Davenport, Iowa. There are now 16 schools in the U.S., from which graduates are joining Health Practitioners in all the modern nations of the world to share healing techniques. Chiropractic is the largest healing profession and benefits millions. Treatment involves soft tissue, spinal and body adjustment to free the nervous system of interferences with normal body function. Its concern is the functional integrity of the musculoskeletal system. In addition to manual methods, chiropractors use physical therapy modalities, exercise, health and nutritional guidance.

F. Mathius Alexander Technique – Lessons intended to end improper use of neuromuscular system and bring body posture back into balance. Eliminates psycho-physical interferences, helps release long-held tension, and aids in re-establishing muscle tone.

Feldenkrais Method – Founded by Dr. Moshe Feldenkrais in the late 1940s. Lessons lead to improved posture and help create ease and efficiency of movement. A great stress removal method.

Caring hands have healing life force energy . . . babies love and thrive with daily massages and cuddles. Family pets love soothing, healing touches. Everyone benefits from healing massages and treatments! – Patricia Bragg

Homeopathy – Dr. Samuel Hahnemann developed homeopathy in the 1800s. Patients are treated with minute amounts of substances similar to those that cause a particular disease to trigger the body's own defenses. The homeopathic principle is *like cures like*. This safe and nontoxic remedy is the #1 alternative therapy in Europe and Britain because it's inexpensive and seldom has any side effects and gets amazing, fast results.

Naturopathy – Brought to America by Dr. Benedict Lust, M.D., this treatment uses diet, herbs, homeopathy, fasting, exercise, hydrotherapy, manipulation and sunlight. (Dr. Paul Bragg was a graduate of Dr. Lust's first Naturopathic School in the U.S.) Practitioners work with your body to restore health naturally. They reject surgery and drugs except as a last resort.

Osteopathy – The first School of Osteopathy was founded in 1892 by Dr. Andrew Taylor Still, M.D. There are now 15 such colleges in the U.S. Treatment involves soft tissue, spinal and body adjustments that free the nervous system from interferences that can cause illness. Healing by adjustment also includes good nutrition, physical therapies, proper breathing and good posture. Dr. Still's premise was that structure and function of the human body are interdependent; if the body structure is altered or abnormal, function is altered and illness results.

242

Reflexology or Zone Therapy – Founded by Eunice Ingham, author of "The Story The Feet Can Tell," whose health career was inspired by a Bragg Health Crusade when she was 17. Reflexology helps the body by removing crystalline deposits from meridians (nerve endings) of the feet through deep pressure massage. A form of Reflexology has its early origins in China and is known to have been practiced by Kenyan natives and North American Indian tribes for centuries. Reflexology helps to activate the body's natural flow of healthy energy by dislodging the collected deposits.

Reiki – A Japanese form of massage that means "Universal Life Energy." Reiki helps the body to detoxify, then rebalance and heal itself. Discovered in the ancient Sutra manuscripts by Dr. Mikso Usui in 1822.

Rolfing – A technique developed by Ida Rolf in the 1930s in the U.S., variously called structural processing, postural release or structural dynamics. It is based on the concept that distortions of normal function of organs and skeletal muscles occur throughout life and are accentuated by the effects of gravity on the body. Rolfing helps the individual to achieve balance and improved body posture. Methods involve the use of stretching, deep tissue massage and relaxation techniques to loosen old injuries and break bad movement and posture patterns, which can cause long-term body stress.

Tragering – Founded by Dr. Milton Trager M.D., who was inspired at age 18 by Paul C. Bragg to become a doctor. It is an experimental learning method that involves gentle shaking and rocking, suggesting a greater letting go, releasing tensions and lengthening of muscles for more body health. Tragering can do miraculous healing where needed in the muscles and the entire body.

Water Therapy – For a great shower, apply almond, avocado, sesame or olive oil to skin, then alternate hot and cold water and massage needed areas while under spray. Garden hose massage is great in summer. Tub baths are wonderful: apply oil and massage. For muscle aches, add 1 cup apple cider vinegar or Epsom salts.

243

Dry Skin Brushing (brush lightly) is wonderful for circulation, toning and healing. For variety use a loofah sponge for massaging in the shower and tub.

Massage – Aromatic – It works two ways: the essence (smell) helps the patient relax as does the massage itself, while the massage is used to help absorption of essential natural oils used for centuries to treat numerous complaints. For example, Tiger Balm, echinacea and arnica help relieve muscle aches. Avoid creams and lotions with mineral oil because it clogs the skin's pores. Almond, avocado and olive oils are good and the most popular. There are over 40 aromatics to use derived from herbs and other botanicals. (Pure rosemary oil, 6 drops to 6 ounces of almond oil, is a favorite.)

Fasting reduces the immune system's workload, increases tissue oxygenation, and releases and excretes fat-stored toxins. – James. F. Balch, M.D.

Massage – Self – Paul C. Bragg often said, "You can be your own best massage therapist, even if you have only one good hand." Near-miraculous improvements have been achieved by victims of accidents or strokes in bringing life back to afflicted parts of their own bodies by self-massage and even vibrators. Treatments can be day or night, almost continual. Also, self-massage can help achieve relaxation at day's end. Families and friends can learn and exchange massages; it's a wonderful sharing experience. Remember, babies also love and thrive with daily massages – start from birth. Your family pets also love the soothing, healing touch of massage.

Massage – Shiatsu – Japanese form of massage that applies pressure from the fingers, hands, elbows and even knees along the same points as acupuncture. Used in Asia for centuries to relieve pain, common ills, muscle stress and to aid lymphatic circulation.

Massage – Sports – An important support system for professional and amateur athletes. Sports massage: improves circulation and mobility to injured tissue, enables athletes to recover more rapidly from myofascial injury, reduces muscle soreness and chronic strain patterns. Soft tissues are freed of trigger points and adhesions, thus contributing to improvement of peak neuro-muscular functioning and athletic performance.

Massage – Swedish – One of the oldest and most-used massage techniques. It's deep body massage that soothes, promotes circulation and is also a great way to loosen and relax muscles before and after exercise.

Author's Comment: My father and I have personally sampled many of these techniques. It's estimated that by the year 2000 U.S. health care costs will reach over $2 trillion. It's more important than ever that we be responsible for our own health. This includes seeking holistic health practitioners who are dedicated to keeping us well by inspiring us to practice prevention! These Alternative Healing Therapies are also popular and getting results – color, aroma, music, biofeedback, Tai Chi, yoga, etc. Explore them and be open to improving your earthly temple for a healthy, happy, longer life. Seek and find the best for your body, mind and soul.

– Patricia Bragg

The heart that loves is always young. – Greek proverb

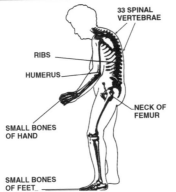

33 SPINAL VERTEBRAE

RIBS

HUMERUS

NECK OF FEMUR

SMALL BONES OF HAND

SMALL BONES OF FEET

OSTEOPOROSIS
Affects 20 Million and Kills 300,000 Americans Annually

Boron
Miracle Trace Mineral For Healthy Bones

BORON – A trace mineral for healthier bones that also helps the body absorb more vital calcium, minerals and necessary hormones! Good sources are most vegetables, fresh and sun-dried fruits, raw nuts, soybeans and nutritional yeast.

The U.S. Department of Agriculture's Human Nutrition Lab in Grand Forks, North Dakota, says boron is usually found in soil and in foods, but many Americans eat a diet low in boron. They conducted a 17 week study which showed that a daily 3 mg. boron supplement enabled participants to reduce the loss (demineralization) of calcium, phosphorus and magnesium from their bodies. This loss is usually caused by eating processed fast foods and lots of meat, salt, sugar and fat and a dietary lack of fresh vegetables, fruits and whole grains.

245

For back and arthritis pain try a glucosamine supplement.

After only 8 weeks on boron, participants' calcium loss was cut 40%. It also helped double the levels of important hormones vital in maintaining calcium and healthy bones. Millions of women on estrogen replacement therapy for osteoporosis may want to use boron as a healthier choice. Also check out the natural progesterone cream from raw yams.*

Scientific studies have shown that women benefit from a healthy lifestyle that includes some gentle sunshine and ample exercise to maintain healthier bones, combined with a low-fat, high-fiber and carbohydrate diet. This helps protect against heart disease, high blood pressure, cancer and many other ailments. I'm happy to see science now agrees with my Dad who first stated these simple health truths over 85 years ago!

* *For more hormone and osteoporosis facts read John Lee, M.D.'s book* What Your Doctor May Not Tell You About Menopause

Miraculous Testimonials
for *The Miracle of Fasting*

These are just a few of the thousands of testimonials we receive yearly, praising fasting for the rejuvenation benefits they reap – physically, mentally and spiritually.

"What a wonderful difference I have felt physically, mentally and, most important to me, spiritually."
– Tully Strong, Coos Bay, OR

"For over 20 years I have been reading the Bragg Books. In fact, *The Miracle of Fasting* saved my life. Your father was a God-sent humanitarian."
– Raymond M. Webster, S.T.D.M., Chicago, Illinois

246

"The results were miraculous! I got rid of a constant cold, and I feel so good and healthy again."
– Nestor R. Villagra, Toronto, Ontario, Canada

"Rock and roll health is better than rock and roll wealth. Thanks to Bragg, the road ain't a drag. We thank the Braggs for the super smooth going on our recent 20 city tour of England."
– David Polemeni, Boy's Town Band, Fort Lee, NJ

"Fasting has helped me clean out my sick body and brain. I feel like a new person. I'm reborn!" – Joe Scavens, SC

"It's great - needs to be reread to get full meaning. Has even helped me with a pinched nerve (7th cervical)."
– Charles A. Aceto, Jr., Winter Park, FL

"I could hardly put it down. Thank you – *The Miracle of Fasting* has thoroughly stirred my inner man."
– Evangelist Richard Sego, Macon, GA

"*The Miracle of Fasting* and *The Bible* are two of my greatest treasures." – Donald G. Smith, Pacifica, CA

Praises for *The Miracle of Fasting*

"As for me and my 'house' I am going to serve the Lord and find my best health through Bragg Health teachings. God knows these are basic truths of nutrition!" – R. Stack

"I'm truly thrilled by what I've read, excited, enthused and confident of newer ways to health."
– Ken Cooper, D.C., Narrabri, NSW, Australia

"I have read *The Miracle of Fasting* more than once. Jesus sure is using you with these wise, beautiful truths that you inspire us to health with."
– Mamie Kostelansky, Monessin, PA

"You've recharged me with hope, encouragement and love which poured from your words. I'm now able to fast without cigarettes and coffee, you've certainly improved my life!"   – Marie Furia, West Orange, NJ

247

"I am eternally grateful for your book. It's made a great difference in my life. I'm sharing it with my friends."
– Carolyn Orrfel, Washington, D.C.

"I live according to the principles you advocate. As a result I am enjoying good health."
– Mark McGinley, M.D., Pietermaritzburg, South Africa

"I have utilized your book's precepts and in turn have reaped overflowing health, joy and energy."
– Gill Contreras, Texarkana, TX

"I thank God and the events in my life for leading me to this book."   – Carol Ann Welch, Cheney, WA

"I have lost all my excess weight with fasting and following your teachings. Now my friends are going to start eating the Bragg way, too." – R. Cortez, Upland, CA

Praises for *The Miracle of Fasting*

"I've experienced a beautiful, remarkable, spiritual awakening. Since reading this book I'll never be quite the same again."   – Sandy Tuttle, Painesville, OH

"Your book gives me so much motivation when I need it. Thank you again for your inspiration, I am honored to be among your many students worldwide."
– John F. Crann, Livingston, NJ

"I am grateful to you and your father's work in writing *The Miracle of Fasting*. I give a copy to each of my patients."
– John M. Leigl, D.C., Racine, Wisconsin

"Our lives have completely turned around! Our family is feeling so healthy and good, we must tell you about it."
– Gene & Joan Zollner, Parents of 11, Bellingham, WA

"Your fasting book has renewed my youth. I'm 58 years young and feel 18. I can outrun 18 year olds! Through your fasting plan, I have lost over 86 pounds and feel a rejuvenated sense of youth."
– Donald Daigh, Key West, FL

   We get letters daily at our Santa Barbara headquarters. We would love to receive testimonials on any of the blessings and healings you have experienced after following The Bragg Healthy Lifestyle with fasting. It's all within your grasp to be in top health. By following this book, you can reap Super Health and a happy, long, vital life! It's never too late to begin – remember the study they did with people in their 80s and 90s! Amazing results were obtained with exercise. You can receive miracles with nutrition, exercise and fasting!

   My love & prayers go out to your heart, mind & soul,

Patricia

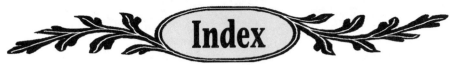

Index

A

Abdomen 113-118, 181, 183-199
Acid crystals 39-46, 62, 201
Acidosis 34-35, 37
Acupuncture 241, 244
Adrenals 168
Air baths 149
Air pollution 7-9, 220
Alcohol 20, 23, 25, 33, 35, 56-57,
   110-111, 119, 170, 191-192
Alkaline 34-38, 44, 85, 221, 238
Allergies 176, 237
Antibiotics 94
Apple Cider Vinegar 23, 38, 75, 161,
   230-231, 238, 244
Arteries 133-138, 168
Arteriosclerosis 37, 95, 134, 164
Arthritis 162, 172, 238, 245
Autointoxication 29-31, 36-37, 56, 181

B

Backache 42, 197-201
Beverages 161, 230, 238
Bible, fasting in 28, 50, 77, 177, 213
Bible quotes 1, 13, 27-28, 32, 145,
   161, 164, 177, 190, 192-193, 202,
   204, 209, 213, 221, 229, 249-251
Bladder 11, 15, 99, 157, 164
Blood 30, 34, 60, 136, 138, 158, 166,
   168, 174, 181, 184-185
Blood pressure 16, 37, 112-113
Bones 41, 115, 155, 166
Bragg Healthy Lifestyle 2, 4-5, 27,
   44, 80, 86, 91, 132, 135, 140, 182,
   198, 219, 230, 238, 248
Brain 57, 169, 203-208
Breathing 6-7, 145-150, 242
Brewer's yeast 78, 93
Brushing, dry skin 243

C

Caffeine 23, 25, 33, 35, 110-111, 163, 191
Calcium 162-163
Cancer 112, 176, 220, 232, 234-235
Carbon dioxide 82, 146, 150-151, 156-157
Cardiovascular 133-138
Cells 48, 156, 178
   in food 172
   inorganic & organic 61
Children 17, 32, 114, 149, 163, 170
Chiropractic 241
Chlorine 8, 14
Chlorophyll 72, 142
Cholesterol 95, 106, 133-138, 235
Chronic fatigue 34, 103, 153
Circulation 154, 168, 189, 244
Cleansing 69, 99
Colds 14, 81, 125-127, 163
Colon 79-80, 87, 103, 156
Constipation 80, 97, 167, 206

D

Dairy products 106, 133, 233, 232
Deficiencies 163, 165, 220
Degenerative diseases 172, 233
Dehydration 109, 156-157, 160
Dental problems 162
Depression 30
Detoxification 86, 123, 210, 235
Digestion 6, 38, 51, 91, 102, 156-157
Doctor Exercise 179-189
Doctor Fasting 177-178
Doctor Fresh Air 145-151
Doctor Good Food 165-177
Doctor Good Posture 197-202
Doctor Human Mind 203-208
Doctor Pure Water 153-164
Doctor Rest 189-196
Doctor Sunshine 141-144
Drugs 23, 30, 33, 80, 110-111, 170, 191, 205

Touch is a primal need, as necessary for growth as a food, clothing or shelter. Michelangelo knew this: when he painted God extending a hand toward Adam on the ceiling of the Sistine Chapel, he chose touch to depict the gift of life. – George H. Colt

---

The Bragg books are written to inspire and guide you to radiant health and longevity. Remember, the book you don't read won't help. So please read and reread the Bragg Books and live The Bragg Healthy Lifestyle!

E

Ears 105
Elimination 51, 67, 80, 87, 90-91, 98, 215
Energy 6, 23, 26, 42,77, 115, 222
Exercise 4, 25, 44, 54-55, 77, 79, 108, 114,
    117-118, 122, 125, 132-133, 140, 145,
    148-149, 153, 165, 168, 179, 181-182,
    183-188, 192, 194, 197-98, 200, 212,
    220, 241-242, 244-245, 248
Eyes 51, 159, 166, 214

F

Fasting 4, 11, 26, 52, 67, 117, 151, 173,
    210, 213, 242
Fatigue 84, 159
Fat 114
Fats 170
Fear 5, 206-207
Fever 7, 107, 125, 159, 204
Fiber 104, 167, 174, 176-177
Fluoride 32, 153
Food allergies 176
Foods 10, 13, 165-177, 224, 235, 238, 232
Foods to Avoid 237
Fruits 35, 55, 57, 93, 163, 225

G

Gastric juices & glands 156
Gastrointestinal tract 91, 105
Glands 99, 168
Goiter 169
Grains 227
Growth stimulators 94

H

Habits 25, 110, 205
Hair 166, 167
Halitosis 84
Hardening of the arteries 162
HDL, Cholesterol 138
Headaches 35, 161, 237
Health care costs 172, 244
Heart 16, 18, 133-135, 153, 168,
    201, 232
    chart 138
Homeopathy 242
Hormones 94, 168
Hunger 36, 215
Hydrogenated fat 106

I

Illness, signs of 159
Inorganic minerals 62
Inorganic salts 158
Insomnia 195-196
Intestinal tract 89, 98, 156-157
Iodine 169

J

Joints 39, 42, 153
Juices 59, 104
Juice fast 58, 230

K

Kelp (Iodine) 169
Kidneys 6, 16, 24, 75, 99, 157, 161

L

Ligaments 197
Liver 99, 103, 156
Longevity 2, 3, 29, 144
Lungs 99, 105, 157

M

Magnesium 162
Massage 154, 242-244
Meat 35, 92-95, 109, 133, 152,
    176, 223, 232
Memory 49, 136
Metabolism 146, 155, 160
Mind 203-208
Mineral supplements 138, 163
Mucus 15, 99, 105-109, 210
Muscles 111, 159, 179-181, 195, 197

N

Naturopathy 242
Nerves 15, 54, 160, 189, 191
Nicotine 110, 112
Nose 99, 157
Nuts & Seeds, chart 225

O

Organic minerals 62
Osteoporosis 163, 245
Overeating 114
Overweight 17, 113
Oxygen 145-151, 156

The good man finds life; the evil man, death. – Proverbs 11:20

P

Pancreas 156, 168
Paraffin wax, deadly 12
Parathyroids 168
Pep Drink 230
Pesticides 9-11
Phosphorus 162
Phytochemicals, chart 235
Pituitary 168
Pneumonia 105
Popcorn recipe 230
Posture 197-201, 241-243
Potassium 163, 236
Practitioners, health 241-244
Premature ageing 45, 129-132, 151
Pressure, therapy 243
Product Summary, chart 232
Proteins 35, 94, 155, 232

R

Rational fasting 105
Rashes 85
Raw food diet 92
Red blood cells 165
Reflexology 242
Reiki 242
Relaxation 190, 194-196, 243
Rice Casserole 231
Rolfing, therapy 243

S

Saliva 157, 161
Salt 14-23, 106, 163, 170
Sedatives 19
Sex glands 168
Shiatsu therapy 244
Skeleton 166, 197
Skin 110, 157-158, 167, 179, 214
Sleep 33, 149, 190-191, 195, 196
Smoking Danger Facts 112
Sodium, natural, in foods 21
Spine 197-201
Starches 35, 79, 121, 138, 156
Stimulants 33, 191-192
Stomach 30, 37, 57, 118, 167
Stress 192
Stretching 243
Sugar 23, 25, 35, 37, 163, 227, 238

Sunshine 141-142, 220, 242
Sweetenings, natural 227
Synovial fluid for joints 39
Systems, body 9, 40, 58, 103, 120, 162, 241-242

T

Tai Chi 244
Teeth 166
Ten-day fast 69
Tension 206
Testimonials 246-248
Therapies 241-244
Thinking 204
Throat 99, 157
Thyroid gland 168-169
Tobacco 23, 25, 33, 110-111, 133, 191
Tomatoes 235
Tongue 97-100
Toxic poison 6, 8-14, 24-27, 67, 85, 103, 157, 170, 174, 191, 210
Tranquilizer, natural 216

U

Underweight 119-123
Urine 22, 75, 95, 106-107, 156, 161

V

Vegetable proteins 226, 233
Vegetables 20, 35, 89, 90, 176, 226, 233
Vegetarian Diet 79, 92-95, 109, 221
Vital Force 6, 12, 40, 56, 75, 103, 107, 125-126, 136, 177, 181
Vitamin D 141-144, 220
Vitamins 138, 164, 167, 234

W

Walking 150, 181, 212
Water 7, 60-66, 75, 153-164
Water fast 5, 11, 22, 26-27, 30, 34, 43-45, 57-58, 75-76, 122
Weight-lifting 185-187

Y

Yoga 244

Z

Zinc 138, 162

Follow the steps of the godly instead, and stay on the right path, for only good men enjoy life to the full. – Proverbs 2:20-21

FROM THE AUTHORS

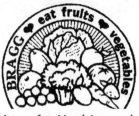

GO ORGANIC

This book was written for You! It can be your passport to a healthy, long, vital life. We in the Alternative Health Therapies join hands in one common objective – promoting a high standard of health for everyone. Healthy nutrition points the way – which is Mother Nature and God's Way. This book teaches you how to work with them, not against them. Health Doctors, therapists nurses, teachers and caregivers are becoming more dedicated than ever to keep their patients healthy and fit. This book was written to speed the spread of this tremendous message of living a healthy lifestyle close to Mother Nature and God.

Statements in this book are scientific health findings, known facts of physiology, biological therapeutics. Paul C. Bragg practiced the natural methods of living for over 80 years with highly beneficial results, knowing that they were safe and of great value. His daughter Patricia Bragg worked with him to carry on the Bragg Health Crusades.

Paul C. Bragg and daughter Patricia express their opinions solely as Public Health Educators and Health Crusaders. They offer no cure for disease. Only the body has the ability to cure a person. Experts may disagree with some of the statements made in this book. However, such statements are considered to be factual, based upon the long-time health experience of pioneer Paul C. Bragg and Patricia Bragg. If you suspect you have a medical problem, please seek alternative health professionals to help you make the healthiest, wisest and best-informed choices.

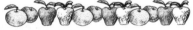

Bragg Blessings to You, Our Treasured Friends

From the Bragg home to yours we share our health knowledge – years of living close to God and Mother Nature. What joys of fruitful, radiant living this produces – this my Father and I want to share with you and your loved ones. With Love and Blessings for Health, Peace and Happiness.

Dear friend, I wish above all things that thou may prosper and be in health even as the soul prospers. – 3 John 2

To maintain good health, normal weight and increase the good life of radiant health, joy and happiness, the body must be exercised properly (stretching, walking, jogging, running, biking, swimming, deep breathing, good posture, etc.) and nourished wisely with natural foods. – Paul C. Bragg

Send for Free Health Bulletins

Let Patricia Bragg send you, your relatives and friends the latest discoveries on Health, Nutrition, Exercise and Longevity. These are sent free periodically. All donations and gifts are tax deductible and appreciated for our spreading the gospel of health to everyone, including schools, churches, prisons and institutions, etc. Also, your donations will help fund our planned Health Retreats which are needed now more than ever! For more information please see page II up front.

With Blessings of Health and Thanks,

Patricia

Please print or type addresses clearly . . .

BRAGG HEALTH CRUSADES, Box 7, Santa Barbara, CA 93102

● _____
Name
_____ ( ) _____
Address   Phone
_____
City   State   Zip Code

● _____
Name
_____ ( ) _____
Address   Phone
_____
City   State   Zip Code

● _____
Name
_____ ( ) _____
Address   Phone
_____
City   State   Zip Code

● _____
Name
_____ ( ) _____
Address   Phone
_____
City   State   Zip Code

● _____
Name
_____ ( ) _____
Address   Phone
_____
City   State   Zip Code

BRAGG ALL NATURAL LIQUID AMINOS

Delicious, Healthy Seasoning Alternative to Tamari & Soy Sauce

BRAGG LIQUID AMINOS – Nutrition you need...taste you will love...a family favorite for over 85 years. A delicious source of nutritious life-renewing protein from soybeans only. Add to or spray over casseroles, soups, sauces, gravies, potatoes, popcorn, and vegetables. An ideal "pick-me-up" broth at work, home or the gym. Gourmet health replacement for Tamari and Soy Sauce. Start today and add more Amino Acids to your daily diet for healthy living – the easy BRAGG LIQUID AMINOS Way!

SPRAY or DASH brings NEW TASTE DELIGHTS! PROVEN & ENJOYED BY MILLIONS.

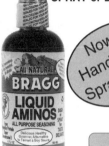

Now in Handy 6 oz Spray Bottle

Spray or Dash of Bragg Aminos Brings New Taste Delights to Season:
- Salads
- Dressings
- Soups
- Veggies
- Tofu
- Rice/Beans
- Tempeh
- Stir-frys
- Wok foods
- Gravies
- Sauces
- Meats
- Poultry
- Fish
- Popcorn
- Casseroles & Potatoes
- Macrobiotics

Pure Soybeans and Pure Water Only
- No Added Sodium
- No Coloring Agents
- No Preservatives
- Not Fermented
- No Chemicals
- No Additives

BRAGG LIQUID AMINOS

SIZE	PRICE	USA SHIPPING & HANDLING	AMT	$ TOTAL
6 oz.	$ 2.98 ea.	Please add $3 for 1st 3 bottles – $1.25 each additional bottle.		•
6 oz.	$ 68.54 Case/24	S/H Cost by Time Zone: CA $5. PST/MST $7. CST $9. EST $11.		•
16 oz.	$ 3.95 ea.	Please add $3 for 1st bottle – $1.25 each additional bottle.		•
16 oz.	$ 43.45 Case/12	S/H Cost by Time Zone: CA $6. PST/MST $7. CST $10. EST $11.		•
32 oz.	$ 6.45 ea.	Please add $4 for 1st bottle – $1.50 each additional bottle.		•
32 oz.	$ 70.95 Case/12	S/H Cost by Time Zone: CA $8. PST/MST $11. CST $16. EST $19.		•

Bragg Liquid Aminos is a food and not taxable

Foreign orders, please inquire on postage

Please Specify: ☐ Check ☐ Money Order ☐ Cash

Charge To: ☐ Visa ☐ MasterCard ☐ Discover

Total Aminos	$ •
Shipping & Handling	•
Total Enclosed (USA Funds Only)	$ •

Credit Card Number: _ _ _ _ _ _ _ _ _ _ _ _ _ _ _ _

Card Expires: Month | Year ___|___

Signature: _____

CREDIT CARD ORDERS ONLY
CALL **(800) 446-1990**
OR FAX **(805) 968-1001**

Business office calls (805) 968-1020. We accept MasterCard Discover or VISA phone orders. Please prepare your order using this order form. It will speed your call and serve as your order record. Hours: 9 am to 4 pm Pacific Time, Monday thru Thursday.
Visit our Web Site: http://www.bragg.com & e-mail: bragg@bragg.com

Mail to: HEALTH SCIENCE, Box 7, Santa Barbara, CA 93102 USA

Please Print or Type – Be sure to give street & house number to facilitate delivery.

A-BOF-806

•
Name

•
Address   Apt. No.

•
City   State

Phone ( )   • Zip

Bragg Aminos – Taste You Love, Nutrition You Need!
Available Health Stores - Nationwide

BRAGG "HOW-TO, SELF-HEALTH" BOOKS

Authored by America's First Family of Health
Live Longer – Healthier – Stronger Self-Improvement Library

Qty.	Bragg Book Titles	ORDER FORM	Health Science ISBN 0-87790	Price	$ Total
_____	Apple Cider Vinegar — Miracle Health System			6.95	•
_____	The Bragg Healthy Lifestyle - Vital Living to 120 (formerly Toxicless Diet)			7.95	•
_____	Super Power Breathing for Super Energy – High Health			7.95	•
_____	Miracle of Fasting (Bragg Bible of Health for physical rejuvenation & longevity)			8.95	•
_____	Water – The Shocking Truth (learn safest water to drink & why)			7.95	•
_____	Nature's Healing System to Improve Eyesight in 90 days (foods, exercises, etc.)			7.95	•
_____	Bragg's Complete Gourmet Recipes for Vital Health – 448 pages			8.95	•
_____	Bragg Health & Fitness Manual – Triathalon Manual – Swim-Bike-Run – for All Ages				•
	A Must for Athletes, Triathletes & would-be-athletes – 600 pages			16.95	•
_____	Build Powerful Nerve Force (reduce stress, fear, anger, worry)			7.95	•
_____	Keep Your Heart & Cardiovascular System Healthy & Fit at Any Age			7.95	•
_____	Nature's Way to Reduce (lose 10 pounds in 10 days)			6.95	•
_____	Hair and Your Health, Nature's Way to Beautiful Hair (easy-to-do method)			7.95	•
_____	Sauerkraut & Cabbage Recipes Raw, Salt-Free (make your own – it's so healthy)			2.95	•
_____	Healthy, Strong Feet – "Best Complete Foot Progam" – Dr. Scholl			7.95	•
_____	Fitness/Spine Motion – For More Flexible, Pain-free Back			3.95	•
_____	Nature's Way to Health (simple method for long, healthy life to 120)			6.95	•

Total Copies Prices subject to change without notice.	**TOTAL BOOKS** $ •
USA Shipping ⟩ Please add $2.00 for first book, $1.00 for each additional book.	**CA residents add sales tax** •
	Shipping & Handling •
USA retail book orders over $35 add $5 only. Canada & Foreign orders add $2.00 per book.	**TOTAL ENCLOSED** $ • (USA Funds Only)

Please Specify: ☐ Money Order ☐ Cash ☐ Check

Charge To: ☐ Visa ☐ Master Card ☐ Discover   Month   Year

Credit Card Number: __ __ __ __ — __ __ __ __ — __ __ __ __ — __ __ __ __   Card Expires: ____|____

[MasterCard] [VISA] [DISCOVER] **Signature:** _____

CREDIT CARD ORDERS ONLY CALL **(800) 446-1990** OR FAX **(805) 968-1001** 🕿	**Business office calls (805) 968-1020.** We accept MasterCard Discover or VISA phone orders. Please prepare your order using this order form. It will speed your call and serve as your order record. Hours: 9 am to 4 pm Pacific Time, Monday thru Thursday. **Visit our Web Site: http://www.bragg.com & e-mail: bragg@bragg.com**

Mail to: **HEALTH SCIENCE, Box 7, Santa Barbara, CA 93102 USA**

Please Print or Type – Be sure to give street & house number to facilitate delivery.

BOF 806

•
_____
Name

•
_____
Address   Apt. No.

•   •
_____   _____
City   State

Phone (_____)   • Zip

Bragg Organic Raw Apple Cider Vinegar
With the Mother . . . Nature's Delicious, Healthy Miracle

HAVE AN APPLE HEALTHY DAY!

– IF ? –

Your Favorite Health Store doesn't carry Bragg Raw Organic Vinegar Ask them to Contact their Health Distributor to stock it! Or they can Call Bragg at 1-800-446-1990

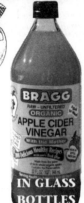

BRAGG
RAW – UNFILTERED
ORGANIC
APPLE CIDER
VINEGAR
With the Mother

IN GLASS BOTTLES

INTERNAL BENEFITS:
- Rich Miracle Enzymes & Potassium
- Natural Antibiotic & Germ Fighter
- Helps Control & Normalize Weight
- Improves Digestion & Assimilation
- Helps Fight Arthritis & Stiffness
- Relieves Sore & Dry Throats
- Helps Remove Toxins & Sludge

EXTERNAL BENEFITS:
- Helps Promote Youthful, Healthy Body
- Helps Promote & Maintain Healthy Skin
- Soothes Sunburn, Shingles & Bites
- Helps Prevent Dandruff & Itchy Scalp
- Soothes, Aching Joints & Muscles

BRAGG ORGANIC APPLE CIDER VINEGAR

SIZE	PRICE	USA SHIPPING & HANDLING	AMT	$ TOTAL
16 oz.	$ 2.19 ea.	Please add $3 for 1st bottle and $1.50 each additional bottle		.
16 oz.	$ 24.09 Case/12	S/H Cost by Time Zone: CA $7. PST/MST $8. CST $12. EST $14.		.
32 oz.	$ 3.79 ea.	Please add $4 for 1st bottle and $2.00 each additional bottle.		.
32 oz.	$ 41.69 Case/12	S/H Cost by Time Zone: CA $10. PST/MST $14. CST $20. EST $24.		.

Bragg Vinegar is a food and not taxable

Foreign orders, please inquire on postage.

Please Specify: ☐ Check ☐ Money Order ☐ Cash

Charge To: ☐ Visa ☐ MasterCard ☐ Discover

Credit Card Number:

Total Vinegar	$.
Shipping & Handling	.
Total Enclosed (USA Funds Only)	$.

Month Year
Card Expires: _____|____

MasterCard   VISA   DISCOVER   **Signature:** _____

Business office calls (805) 968-1020. We accept MasterCard Discover or VISA phone orders. Please prepare your order using this order form. It will speed your call and serve as your order record. Hours: 9 am to 4 pm Pacific Time, Monday thru Thursday.
Visit our Web Site: http://www.bragg.com & e-mail: bragg@bragg.com

Mail to: **HEALTH SCIENCE, Box 7, Santa Barbara, CA 93102 USA**

Please Print or Type – Be sure to give street & house number to facilitate delivery.

V-BOF-806

Name _____

Address _____ Apt. No. _____

City _____ State _____

Phone (___) _____ • Zip _____

Bragg Apple Cider Vinegar – Taste You Love, Health You Need!
Available Health Stores - Nationwide